FOOD & FITNESS

JAN NIX

AND

LINDA CARLSON, R.D.

HPBooks

Published by HPBooks, a division of Price Stern Sloan, Inc.
360 North La Cienega Boulevard, Los Angeles, California 90048
©Copyright HPBooks 1988
1st Printing

NOTICE: The information contained in this book is true and complete to the best of our knowledge. All recommendations are made without any guarantees on the part of the authors or HPBooks. The authors and publisher disclaim all liability in connection with the use of this information.

Nix, Jan.
    Food & fitness/Jan Nix and Linda Carlson.
      p.   cm.
    Includes index.
    ISBN 0-89586-622-6
    1. Nutrition. 2. Diet. 3. Health. 4. Physical fitness.
I. Carlson, Linda (Linda Kay)   II. Title.   Title: Food and fitness.
RA784.N58 1988   88-4992
641.5′63—dc19   CIP

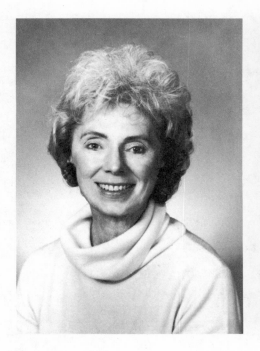 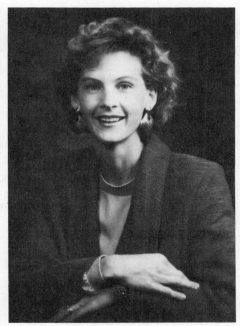

Jan Nix and Linda Carlson

Both *Jan Nix* and *Linda Carlson* are eminently qualified to be the authors of *Food & Fitness*. They both practice the guidelines for good health that are outlined in this book. **Jan Nix,** with a degree in home economics, has experience in teaching, editing and developing recipes, and has several cookbooks to her credit. She has taught a wide range of cooking classes—from basic cooking to the intricacies of Japanese cuisine that she learned while living in Japan. A veteran traveler Jan lives with her family in Northern California, where she takes advantage of the many outdoor experiences available. She enjoys camping, hiking and bicycling.

    Linda Carlson is a Registered Dietitian in private practice who helps individuals maximize their physical health by establishing positive exercise and eating habits. Her clients include fitness labs, businesses with employee wellness programs and running clinics as well as private individuals. Linda attended college on a track scholarship. She competed in track and field for over 13 years. Current interests include running, skiing, swimming and golf. Linda lives with her family in Colorado where she takes a active role in community affairs.

CONTENTS

INTRODUCTION

Food & Fitness is for everyone who wants to eat healthy, good tasting food—from the serious recreational athlete to those who simply want to enjoy a better quality of life. It is for the conscientious individual who wants to live life to the fullest. This book offers information on how much and what kind of food you need to perform at your best. For the athlete, it explains what to eat before and after competition, and what special techniques can enhance performance. This book not only tells you what kinds of food to eat, but how to prepare them. It translates the latest nutrition information into delicious, easy-to-prepare meals.

This book is for the active person who wants to eat nutritious meals without spending all day in the kitchen. Many of the recipes are good enough for company, yet not too elaborate for spur-of-the-moment entertaining. They are simple to prepare if you keep a hectic schedule, yet varied enough to make meals interesting.

As an active person, you have a vital interest in keeping your body running at its best. That means eating right—the right foods in the right amounts. But how do you do that? How do you sort out nutritional fact from fiction? How do you turn good intentions into real food and a regular exercise program?

This book is designed to get you on the road to a healthier lifestyle. Whether you are already exercising and want to know how to maximize your performance by eating correctly, or if you want to start an exercise program for the first time—jump right in. If you are a little overweight and want to know how to lose a few pounds in spite of your hectic lifestyle—this book is for you. These recipes bridge the gap between know how and how to.

Regardless of your activity level, consider the following suggestions for improving your diet:

1. Eat the right number of calories to maintain your ideal weight.
2. Decrease fat and cholesterol.
3. Eat a variety of lightly processed foods.

CALORIES

A calorie is a unit used to measure energy. We get energy primarily from three sources—carbohydrate, fat and protein. Not only does food supply these fuels, but your body can also convert its own stores of carbohydrate, fat and protein into energy. Carbohydrates and proteins contribute 4 calories of energy per gram, while fats have over twice that amount at 9 calories per gram.

Most of your calories, 50 to 55 percent, should come from carbohydrates such as bread, cereal, fruit and starchy vegetables. Twelve to fifteen percent of your calories should come from protein foods like meat, fish, poultry and eggs. No more than 30 percent of your total calories should come from fat such as butter, margarine and oils.

To estimate approximately how many calories and how much carbohydrate, protein and fat you should be eating each day, fill in the blanks of the following equations. First you must determine the number of calories that you need.

CALORIES:
Take your present weight and multiply it by 15 if you are moderately active and 17 if you are very active.

_____ (Your weight) x 15 or 17 = ____ (Daily caloric requirement (DCR))

CARBOHYDRATE (CHO):

_____ (DCR) x 55% = _____ cal from CHO ÷ 4 calories/gram of CHO = _____ grams of CHO per day

FAT:

_____ (DCR) x 30% = _____ cal from fat ÷ 9 calories/gram of fat = _____ grams of fat per day

PROTEIN:

_____ (DCR) x 15% = _____ cal from fat ÷ 4 calories/gram = _____ grams of protein per day

Now that you know the amount of carbohydrate, protein and fat that you need each day, how does that translate into real food? For instance, how many glasses of milk and pieces of chicken can you eat before your protein requirement is used up?

The best way to visualize grams of food is to group foods together that have a similar nutrient content. For example, bread and pasta are grouped together because a serving of each contains about 15 grams of carbohydrate and 2 grams of protein. One ounce of lean meat and 1 egg have about 7 grams of protein and 5 grams of fat and are grouped together. These food groups are exchange lists and are helpful in determining how many servings of each food group you need. See the exchange lists on pages 199-201 or follow the 2-2-4-4 good eating plan.

A DEFINITION OF ACTIVITY LEVELS

SEDENTARY: Little exertion beyond basic activity. If you have a desk job and are sitting or reclining most of the day, you are sedentary.

MODERATELY ACTIVE: Exertion beyond basic activity; occasional bursts of heavier activity. For instance, if you have a desk job, but are on your feet a lot, and exercise 3 to 4 times a week, you are moderately active.

VERY ACTIVE: Constant, intense activity. If you are on your feet much of the time and engage in a strenuous aerobic exercise 6 to 7 days a week, you are very active.

A MORE PRECISE WAY TO ASSESS CALORIC NEEDS

For A Woman:

1) Estimate your ideal weight: use the figure of 100 pounds as a base. Add 5 pounds for every inch above 5 feet. For instance, if you are 5 feet 5 inches tall, use the 100 as a base figure and add 5 x 5, for a total of 125 pounds. This number, give or take 10 percent depending on frame size, is considered your ideal weight.

2) To determine caloric requirement: take your ideal body weight and multiply it by the activity factors listed below:

10 = no activity
13 = sedentary
15 = moderately active
17 = very active

For example, if you are 5 feet 5 inches tall and moderately active, you would need 1875 calories each day to maintain your ideal weight. (125 pounds x 15 = 1875).

For A Man:

1) Estimate your ideal weight: use the figure of 106 pounds as a base. Add 6 pounds for every inch above 5 feet. For instance, if you are 5 feet 10 inches tall, use the 106 as a base figure and add 6 x 10, for a total of 166 pounds. This number, give or take 10 percent depending on frame size, is considered your ideal weight.

2) To determine caloric requirement: take your ideal body weight and multiply it by the activity factors listed below:

10 = no activity
13 = sedentary
15 = moderately active
17 = very active

For example, if your ideal weight is 166 pounds and you are moderately active, you would need about 2500 calories a day (166 x 15 = 2490 calories).

GUIDE TO GOOD EATING

FOOD GROUP	RECOMMENDED NUMBER OF SERVINGS	
	TEENS	**ADULTS** (men and women*)

DAIRY PRODUCTS
    1 serving is
    equivalent to:
1 cup milk or yogurt
1 cup milk-based pudding
1-3/4 cups ice cream
1-1/2 cups low-fat
    cottage cheese
	4	2*

PROTEIN FOODS
    1 serving is
    equivalent to:
3 oz. cooked lean meat,
    fish or poultry
2 eggs
2 oz. cheese
1 cup dried beans, peas
    or lentils, cooked
3 tablespoons peanut butter
	2	2

FRUIT & VEGETABLES
    1 serving is
    equivalent to:
1/2 cup cooked or raw
    vegetables
1 medium-sized piece
    fresh fruit
    1/2 cup juice
	4	4

GRAINS & CEREALS
    1 serving is
    equivalent to:
1 enriched bread slice
1 cup ready-to-eat
    cereal (fortified)
1/2 cup cooked cereal
1/2 cup pasta or rice
	4	4

Adapted from Guide to Good Eating, National Dairy Council
* Pregnant women need 4 servings from the dairy group.

At the very least, you should have 2 to 3 servings of dairy products, 2 (3-ounce) servings of protein foods, 4 servings of bread and cereal and 2 servings each of fruits and vegetables. This is often called the 2-2-4-4 plan. (See chart opposite.)

CALORIES FOR ATHLETES

The 2-2-4-4 eating guide outlined above provides 1200 to 1500 calories, which is fine for the average adult. An athlete, however, needs more calories—about 1000 more per day. Active women should eat a minimum of 1800 to 2000 calories, while a man needs 2500 to 3000 calories a day. Your extra calories can come from any of the exchange lists, just make sure you are getting a good variety of foods. If you are interested in having an individualized menu plan formulated especially for you, see your local registered dietitian.

A low-calorie diet is especially harmful for active women. My good friend and nationally-ranked runner, Julie, is constantly trying to gain that competitive edge. She tries to decrease her percentage of body fat by cutting back drastically on calories, yet she manages to maintain a strenuous training schedule. She is literally running on empty, which can upset the hormonal balance and play a role in the occurrance of amenorrhea (failure to menstruate) common among female athletes. Whether you are male or female, be sure you are eating enough calories to perform at your best.

CARBOHYDRATES

Besides extra calories, an active person needs to eat more carbohydrates. Carbohydrates are divided into two groups—starches and sugars. Sugars are referred to as simple carbohydrates and the starches are called complex carbohydrates. Simple carbohydrates are in foods such as pie, cake, cookies, syrup, jam, jelly, molasses, fruit and table sugar.

Starches or complex carbohydrates are in foods such as breads and cereals, potatoes, rice, pasta, peas, corn and dried beans. These complex carbohydrates should provide at least half of your total calories for each day.

CARBOS FOR GO POWER

The primary function of carbohydrates is to supply energy for your body. Muscles prefer carbohydrate over fat or protein because it is more readily available and "burns" completely unlike fat and protein. Carbohydrate is stored in the form of glycogen, both in the liver and in muscle. If carbohydrate is not available, your body will break down fat and protein for energy. Burning protein for energy is like using your dining room furniture as firewood—it is very expensive! Burning carbohydrate for energy, however, is like using pine logs to fuel a fire. It is more available and much less costly.

In addition to carbohydrate, your body will also burn fat for energy during exercise. A general rule of thumb is: in any activity that lasts less than one minute the body will use primarily carbohydrate for energy. If the activity is longer than one minute, the body begins to burn a mixture of both fat and carbohydrate.

Although your body runs better when it burns carbohydrates for energy, eating only carbohydrates at a meal is not healthy. Many of my clients complain of dizziness and extreme fatigue after eating a high-carbohydrate meal on an empty stomach. This is a fairly common reaction, and can be avoided by eating four to six small meals throughout the day instead of one or two very large meals. Including a small amount of lean protein along with the carbohydrate at each meal is another way to avoid this drop in energy level.

In addition to diet, training plays an important role in the way you burn carbohydrates. Training increases the amount of glycogen your muscles can store. Theoretically, the more glycogen you can store, the more energy that is available for exercise.

SUGAR

Both simple and complex carbohydrates provide energy but, foods containing mostly sugar provide very few calories per nutrient. If you are watching your waistline, every calorie you eat should be packed with nutrients. To trim those "empty" calories from your diet, try some of the following tips:

SUGAR CONTENT IN COMMON FOODS

COMMON FOODS	TEASPOONS OF SUGAR
BEVERAGES	
Root Beer (8 oz.)	3-2/3
Cola drinks (8 oz.)	6
Ginger Ale (8 oz.)	4-1/2
Kool-Aid (8 oz.)	6
CAKES & COOKIES	
Angel food (1/6th of 10-inch cake)	7
Cheesecake (1/8th of 8-inch cake)	2
Chocolate cake with icing (1/6th of 9-inch-square cake)	10
Coffeecake (1/6th of 8-inch-square cake)	3
Brownies, plain (2″ x 2″ x 1″ piece)	3
Oatmeal cookie (2 inches in diameter—1)	2
Doughnut, glazed (1)	6
CANDY	
Milk chocolate bar (1-1/2 oz.)	2-1/2
Chewing Gum (1 stick)	1/2
Fudge (1 oz. square)	4-1/2
Marshmallow (1)	1-1/2
DAIRY PRODUCTS	
Ice cream (3/4 cup)	3-1/2
Ice cream sundae (2 scoops ice cream, 2 tablespoons syrup)	7
Malted milkshake (10 oz.)	5
DESSERTS	
Apple cobbler (1/2 cup)	3
Jell-O gelatin dessert (1/2 cup)	4-1/2
Apple pie (1/8th of 9-inch pie)	7
JAMS, JELLIES, SAUCES	
Jelly (1 tablespoon)	1-1/2
Maple syrup (1 tablespoon)	2-1/2
Honey (1 tablespoon)	3
Chocolate sauce (1 tablespoon)	4-1/2
CANNED FRUIT & JUICE	
Canned fruit juices, sweetened (1/2 cup)	2
Fruit cocktail (1/2 cup)	5
Canned peaches (2 halves with 2 tablespoons syrup)	3-1/2

Adapted from values from the U.S. Department of Agriculture, the American Dental Association and the American Dietetic Association.

• Substitute 1/4 cup of nonfat dry milk powder for 1/4 cup of sugar when baking cakes or muffins. The milk adds some sweetness, but it also adds protein, calcium and riboflavin.

• Don't treat dessert as a final act to every meal. If dinner for you is not dinner without dessert, try a slice of angel food cake or sponge cake topped with fresh fruit or canned fruit packed in its own juice.

• When using less sugar in baking, increase spices, such as cinnamon, nutmeg and allspice. Add extra flavorings, such as vanilla and almond extract.

• Limit your intake of soft drinks, sweetened beverages and sweetened alcohol mixes. Fruit juice, club soda, dry wine, seltzer water or low-fat milk are better choices.

Are some sweeteners better for you than others? Probably not. Molasses, brown sugar, honey and raw sugar all contain sucrose, and are metabolized in the same way as table sugar. The nutrient content of these other sweeteners is negligible. Although they sound healthier, they still contain mostly simple sugars.

WHAT ABOUT ARTIFICIAL SWEETENERS?

The most common artificial sweeteners, Saccharin and Aspartame, are used in a variety of food products from soft drinks to cereals. They add sweetness without the unwanted calories.

Large doses of Saccharin have been linked to cancer in laboratory animals, but it is still allowed on the market with a warning label. Aspartame (marketed as Nutrasweet) is approved for both table-top use and use in beverages and some commercial products. It decomposes with heat, so is not suitable for baking.

In moderation, artificial sweeteners are probably fine, and may serve an important role for the morbidly obese and diabetic individual. I don't usually recommend artificial sweeteners for a healthy normal-weight person, and instead suggest acquiring a taste for less sweet foods, or learning to enjoy the natural sweetness in food.

FIBER

Fiber, found in plant foods, is made up of complex carbohydrates. It is important to your diet because it may reduce the risk of colon cancer and help regulate blood cholesterol levels. The National Cancer Institute recommends a person eat 20 to 30 grams of dietary fiber every day.

MENU WITH APPROXIMATELY 20 GRAMS OF FIBER

	DIETARY FIBER (in grams)
BREAKFAST	
1-1/2 cups Raisin Bran cereal	4.0
1 whole-wheat bread slice	2.1
1/2 small banana	1.5
1 cup skim milk	0
LUNCH	
Roast beef sandwich	
3 oz. lean roast beef	0
2 whole-wheat bread slices	4.2
6 carrot sticks	0.8
1 celery stalk	0.7
1 medium-size peach with skin	3.0
DINNER	
3 oz. roasted chicken (1/2 breast)	0
1 cup green beans	4.0
1/2 cup long-grain white rice	0.8
1 whole-wheat roll	0.8
1 cup fresh strawberries	3.0
SNACK	
2 cups unbuttered popped, popcorn	0.8
TOTAL	24.2 grams

FIBER CONTENT OF COMMON FOODS

APPROXIMATE GRAMS OF DIETARY FIBER

BREADS/CEREALS/PASTA

1/3 cup All Bran cereal	9
1 cup whole wheat pasta, cooked	5
1 medium Bran muffin	3
1 slice whole wheat bread	2
1/3 cup uncooked oatmeal	2
1 cup popped popcorn	2
1 slice white bread	1
1 cup cooked pasta	1

FRUITS/NUTS

1/4 cup almonds	5
3 dried prunes	4
1 medium apple, with skin	3
1 cup strawberries, fresh	3
1 medium banana	3
1 medium orange, fresh	3

VEGETABLES/COOKED LEGUMES

1/2 cup cooked kidney beans	9
1/2 cup cooked pinto beans	5
1/2 cup cooked frozen peas	4
1 medium baked potato, with skin	4
1/2 cup cooked corn	3
1/2 cup cooked broccoli	3
1/2 cup raw cabbage	2
1/2 cup lentils	2
1/2 cup lettuce	1

Adapted from Pennington, Jean and Church, Helen. *Food Values of Portions Commonly Used.* 14th Edition, Harper & Row: New York. 1985.

The different types of dietary fiber contribute different health benefits. Insoluble fiber may reduce the risk of colon cancer and relieves constipation. It is found in whole grains and vegetables. The other type of fiber—soluble fiber may help regulate blood cholesterol; it is found in oatmeal, citrus fruits, apples and dried beans. To relieve constipation, eat whole grain products or high-fiber foods such as wheat bran, broccoli, cabbage, peas or spinach. To lower elevated blood cholesterol, eat a diet high in oat products, dried beans and citrus fruit.

Keep the following suggestions in mind when increasing your fiber intake:
- Gradually increase fiber consumption to avoid intestinal discomfort.
- Keep your fiber intake below 35 grams a day. Too much fiber can interfere with the absorption of some nutrients, such as calcium, iron, magnesium, zinc and copper.
- Eat a variety of high-fiber foods—don't rely on one or two foods for your total fiber intake.

FAT IN YOUR DIET

Dietary fat—the fat found in the food you eat—is important for the active person because of its role in energy production. Fat provides power for the muscles when other forms of energy are depleted. It transports the fat-soluble vitamins, insulates vital organs and makes skin soft and supple. The problem is that the average person eats too much fat. Most of us eat at least 10 percent more fat than we should each day.

Nutritionists are concerned about fat intake because of its correlation with heart disease and cancer. By eating less fat, we can substantially reduce the risk of developing breast, colon and prostate cancer.

Where does fat come from and just how much should we eat each day? The average American eats about 40 percent of his total calories in the form of fat. The American Heart Association recommends that no more than 30 percent of a person's total calories should come from fat. Of that 30 percent, approximately 10 percent should come from saturated fat, 10 percent from monounsaturated and 10 percent from polyunsaturated fat.

SATURATED VERSUS UNSATURATED FAT

Saturation simply describes the chemical composition of a fat. One way to tell the difference between saturated and unsaturated fat is that saturated fat is usually solid at room temperature. For example: lard, butter and the fat around meat all contain saturated fat. Although saturated fat comes primarily from animal sources, there are two vegetable oils that are saturated—coconut oil and palm oil. Both oils are commonly found in commercially prepared food. Too much saturated fat in the diet can increase blood cholesterol and increase your chance for heart attack.

Oils that have been hydrogentated (changed from a liquid to a solid) are also saturated. Read labels on prepared foods to see if the oils have been hydrogenated. Two examples of hydrogenated fat are solid vegetable shortening and most margarines.

Unsaturated fat usually is liquid at room temperature and comes from vegetable sources such as corn, sunflower, safflower and soybean oil. Unsaturated fats tend to lower blood cholesterol.

Monounsaturated fats are found in foods such as olive oil, avocados, peanuts, peanut butter and cashews. Recent studies suggest that monounsaturated fats may also be effective in lowering blood cholesterol levels. Further research is needed before nutritionists recommend a diet high in olive or peanut oil.

A physically active person is not immune to the health risks associated with a high-fat diet. Even a well-conditioned athlete should limit the quantity and type of fat he or she eats. That is why most of the recipes in this book are limited to no more than 15 grams of fat for an entree and 10 grams of fat for a side dish. Not only are the recipes lower in total fat, but they also contain less saturated fat.

If you exercise, your chances of developing coronary heart disease are probably greatly reduced due to the positive lifestyle habits associated with exercise. For example, an athlete rarely smokes, is usually lean and relieves a tremendous amount of stress through exercise. These habits undoubtedly improve a person's quality of life and decrease the chance of having a heart attack. Some risk factors, such as your age or family history, are impossible to change. The important thing is to do something about the risk factors you can change, such as diet and exercise.

Fats are sometimes hard to identify. One of my patients, Jim, was trying to lose weight by eating "diet" foods like cottage cheese, soup, chicken and fish. What Jim didn't realize was that even "diet" foods can be high in fat. A typical day for Jim included foods such as: whole milk, whole-milk cottage cheese, 3 tablespoons salad dressing and a fried chicken sandwich. Jim's "low-fat" diet adds up to 103 grams of fat or 54 percent of his total calories. Become aware of where fats are found.

● Obvious sources: oils, butter, margarine, salad dressing, shortening and lard

● Less obvious sources: pie crust, croissants, fried foods, chips, buttery crackers and doughnuts

● Hidden sources: olives, avocados, whole-milk cheese, tender cuts of red meat, fish and poultry skin, ice cream, nuts, candy, pastries and chocolate.

Some ideas for low-fat meals are included below:

BREAKFAST: 1. Whole-wheat toast with reduced-calorie margarine and orange juice.
2. Oatmeal, Shredded Wheat cereal or Cheerios cereal with low-fat or skim milk and sliced fresh fruit
3. Low-fat yogurt or skim milk with fresh banana and ice cubes blended together into a breakfast shake

LUNCH: 1. 3/4 cup water-packed tuna mixed with low-fat yogurt or reduced calorie mayonnaise on whole-wheat bread

DINNER:
2. Bean tostada with lettuce and tomato
3. Broth-based soup

1. 4 to 5 ounces broiled fish or poultry without skin
2. Stir-fried beef and vegetables with rice
3. Curried Turkey Salad, page 158
4. Eggplant Lasagna, page 133

SUGGESTIONS

To reduce fat in your own diet, try the following suggestions:

• Learn to read labels. Even though a food is labeled low in cholesterol, it still may be high in saturated fat. The term "hydrogenated" will signal that an unsaturated vegetable oil is chemically changed to become saturated. For example: A tablespoon of hydrogenated vegetable shortening contains no cholesterol, yet contains 3.5 grams of saturated fat.

• Avoid whole milk and whole-milk products; use low-fat or skim milk. Use low-fat cheeses such as farmer's, part-skim mozzarella, ricotta and cottage cheese.

• When red meat is eaten, reduce the portion size. Use a lean meat trimmed of all visible fat; broil, bake, roast or barbecue meat until it is at least medium done.

• Cook food in wine, broth, water or flavored vinegar, or use a nonstick pan. Avoid sautéeing in butter, hydrogenated margarine, shortening or lard.

• Use soft tub-style margarine instead of butter or stick margarine. Make sure the first ingredient on the label is a liquid vegetable oil.

• Reduce whole egg consumption.

• Avoid high-fat meats such as bacon, sausage and most luncheon meat.

• Remove fat from meat drippings and broths before using.

• Use convenience foods and commercially baked goods in moderation.

• Include more fish in your diet.

• Plan at least 2 non-meat meals a week. Include a vegetable protein or a pasta dish for variety.

• Dilute bottled salad dressings with lemon juice or vinegar.

• Avoid commercially prepared products that contain palm oil, coconut oil or hydrogenated vegetable oil.

CHOLESTEROL CONTROVERSY

Studies show that eating too much cholesterol may increase blood cholesterol

TYPE OF FAT	FOOD SOURCE	EFFECT ON THE BODY
1. Unsaturated fat	Vegetable foods such as corn oil, safflower oil, sunflower oil, sesame oil, soybean oil, cottonseed oil	Lowers blood cholesterol
2. Monunosaturated fat	Primarily plant foods, such as olive oil and peanut oil	*Neither raises or lowers blood cholesterol
3. Saturated fat	Animal foods such as red meat, whole milk, whole-milk products, cheese, coconut oil, palm oil	Raises blood cholesterol

*Recent studies suggest that monounsaturated fat may be beneficial in lowering blood cholesterol.

Generally speaking, we should increase the amount of unsaturated fat we eat, and decrease the amount of saturated fat and cholesterol we eat.

FAT COUNTDOWN

FOOD	GRAMS OF FAT
PROTEIN	
Ground beef, regular (4 oz.)	36
Ground beef, lean (4 oz.)	23
Steak, sirloin, untrimmed (5 oz.)	49
Spare ribs (4 oz.)	44
Frankfurter, beef or pork	15
Bacon (3 slices)	17
Beef bologna (2 oz.)	13
Poultry, with skin (4 oz.)	8
Poultry, without skin (4 oz.)	4
Egg (1 large)	1-5
Fish, cod, flounder and halibut	0.5
Fish, salmon, trout (4 oz.)	11
Tuna, packed in oil (4 oz.)	13
Tuna, packed in water (4 oz.)	1
DAIRY PRODUCTS	
Ricotta cheese (2 tablespoons)	4
Neufchâtel cheese (2 tablespoons)	7
Cream cheese (2 tablespoons)	10
American cheese (1 oz.)	9
Cheddar cheese (1 oz.)	10
Whole milk (1 cup)	9
Low-fat yogurt (1 cup)	5
BREADS/CEREALS	
Biscuit (2″ diameter)	5
Crackers, buttery type (5)	5
Pancake or waffle (2″ diameter)	5
Potatoes, French-fried (8)	10
Potato or corn chips (15)	10
FATS	
Avocados (1/2)	15
Peanut butter (2 tablespoons)	16
Almonds (24 nuts)	16
Vegetable oil (1 tablespoon)	14
Heavy cream (2 tablespoons)	11
Sour cream (2 tablespoons)	5
Butter (1 tablespoon)	12
Margarine (1 tablespoon)	12
Mayonnaise (1 tablespoon)	11
Italian dressing, bottled, (2 tablespoons)	18
Olives (5 small)	5
DESSERTS	
Ice cream (1/2 cup)	7-12
Frozen yogurt (1/2 cup)	3
Cheesecake (1/8th of 8-inch cake)	14
Pecan pie (1/8th pie)	23
Apple pie (1/8th pie)	12
Cookie (2″ diameter)	3
Sherbet (1/2 cup)	2

Adapted from USDA Handbooks 4, 5 and 6, and 8.

FAT SAVINGS CHART

IN PLACE OF......	GRAMS OF FAT	SUBSTITUTE......	GRAMS OF FAT
Potato chips—(12 chips)	10	Pretzels (25 sticks)	1
Peanuts (1/4 cup)	18	Popcorn, plain (1 cup)	0
Buttery crackers (5)	5	Rye cracker (4-1/2)	0
Cinnamon Danish (1)	7	Bagel (1)	1
Croissant (1)	6	English muffin (1)	1
Whole milk (1 cup)	8	Low-fat milk (1 cup)	4
Whole milk (1 cup)	8	Skim milk (1 cup)	0
Ice cream (1/2 cup)	7	Ice milk (1/2 cup)	2
Yogurt (1 cup whole milk)	7	Low-fat yogurt (1 cup)	4
Milk chocolate bar (1)	10	Granola bar (1 bar)	4
Beef frank (1)	13.5	Turkey frank (1)	8
Round steak, untrimmed (3 oz.)	13	Round steak trimmed	5
Chicken, dark meat with skin (3 oz.)	13	Chicken, dark meat without skin	8
Chicken, breast with skin (3 oz.)	8	Chicken, breast without skin	5
Tuna, light, in oil, drained (3 oz.)	10	Tuna, light, in water, drained	1

Reprinted from *Nutrition Action Healthletter,* which is available from the Center for Science in the Public Interest, 1501 16th Street, NW, Washington, D.C. 20036, for $19.95 for 10 issues. Copyright 1988.

CHOLESTEROL CONTENT OF COMMON FOODS

	CHOLESTEROL (mg.)
MEAT (3 ounces)	
Calf liver, fried	394
Veal and pork	80-86
Lean beef	56
Chicken (light meat)	76
Chicken (dark meat)	82
Egg (1)	274
DAIRY FOODS (1 cup; cheeses, 1 oz.)	
Ice cream	59
Whole milk	33
Butter (1 tablespoon)	31
Yogurt (low-fat)	11
Cheddar cheese	30
American cheese	27
Camembert cheese	20
Parmesan cheese	8
OILS (1 tablespoon)	
Vegetable oils	0
FISH (3 ounces)	
Squid	153
Fish	59
Shrimp (6 large)	48
Clams (6 large)	36

Adapted from Pennington, Jean, and Church, Helen. *Food Values of Portions Commonly Used.* 14th Edition, Harper & Row: New York. 1985.

levels. Elevated blood cholesterol is correlated with an increased incidence of coronary heart disease. A number of factors—age, gender, family history, smoking, exercise and diet influence our cholesterol levels. Most nutritionists recognize the correlation between diet and coronary heart disease and are concerned with a person's total fat intake—not just his cholesterol intake.

In light of this current thinking, animal products, which are big contributors of cholesterol to the diet, are acceptable in moderation. One recommendation by the American Heart Association is to limit cholesterol to 100 mg per 1000 calories per day. The daily maximum should not exceed 300 mg. A diet rich in saturated fat and cholesterol is identified as a major risk factor for coronary heart disease. Remember the following two principles:

• A diet high in saturated fat will raise the cholesterol level of the blood.

• A high blood cholesterol level will increase the risk of coronary heart disease and heart attack.

PROTEIN

Protein is important for the growth and repair of body tissue. It is an essential part of your muscles, skin, connective tissues, hormones and enzymes. The protein you eat keeps all your complex systems in good repair. Protein is made up of building blocks called amino acids. There are 24 of these building blocks, 8 of which are not manufactured by the body and are called essential amino acids. These eight essential amino acids must be provided by the foods that you eat. Meat, poultry, fish and eggs are considered complete proteins because they contain all eight essential amino acids. Other foods such as vegetables and grains contain some of the essential amino acids, but not all eight. Vegetables and grains must be combined with other foods to make them complete.

This combination of complementary proteins is the way vegetarians get enough high quality protein. Ovo-lacto vegetarians—those that eat both eggs and milk products—have no problem getting enough complete protein. Vegetarians who eat only plant products, however,

must make a special effort to combine complementary proteins correctly. The following chart shows how to combine plant protein to make them complete:

GRAINS + LEGUMES: For example, a peanut butter sandwich on whole wheat bread, red beans and rice or a bean tostada made with a corn tortilla and dried beans.

NUTS + GRAINS: For example, granola made with rolled oats, almonds and sunflower seeds.

GRAINS + MILK PRODUCTS: For example, grilled cheese sandwich, macaroni and cheese, cereal with milk, or a rice-cheese casserole.

NUTS + LEGUMES: For example, a snack mixture that contains peanuts and sunflower seeds, or sesame seeds sprinkled on top of a casserole made with beans.

A good source of plant protein is tofu or soybean curd. It has a very mild flavor and it usually takes on the flavor of the food with which it is cooked. Slice or crumble tofu and add it to any spicy dish such as soups, casseroles, salads, stir-fry dishes, dips or spreads. Tofu is a complete protein only when it is combined with a grain such as rice, barley or wheat. It is a good meat substitute because it is low in saturated fat and cholesterol-free.

MEAT-FREE IS NOT NECESSARILY FAT-FREE

If you choose to avoid red meat because of the fat and cholesterol, make sure you are not eating other foods that contain a lot of fat. Be consistent with your dietary objective. Many vegetarians regularly eat eggs, casseroles laden with cheese and nuts. These foods add a substantial amount of fat to the diet. Some guidelines to help vegetarians avoid excessive fat intake are included below:

• Use low-fat cheese, such as farmer cheese or part-skim mozzarella.

• Substitute egg whites for whole eggs when possible in cooking.

• Limit the amount of butter or oil used in sautéeing vegetables.

• Incorporate tofu in the place of meat for casseroles and stir-fry dishes.

• Use peanut butter in moderation.

THE MEAT OF THE MATTER

Red meat—beef, veal, pork and lamb, make an important contribution to a balanced diet. Meat is best known for its high protein content, but it is also high in the B vitamins and iron. In fact, red meat is the best source of vitamin B_{12}, which is usually lacking in a vegetarian diet.

Red meat is also high in iron, most of which is heme iron. Heme iron, found in animal foods, is better utilized by the body than the non-heme iron found in vegetables. Many green vegetables contain substances called oxalates which bind with non-heme iron and prevent its absorption by the body. For instance, only 3 percent of the iron found in spinach is actually absorbed and used by the body. To increase the amount of non-heme iron you absorb, eat a red meat along with vegetables or cereals.

One drawback to red meat is its fat content. Fortunately, red meat is coming to the consumer much leaner than ever before. Pork has about half the fat it did 10 years ago. Lamb is 10 percent leaner.

The various types of red meat differ in the amount of saturated fat they contain. Lean pork and veal contain about 25 percent saturated fat, lean beef has 35 to 45 percent and lamb is about 50 percent saturated. To minimize the amount of saturated fat you get from red meat, reduce highly processed types of meat like sausage, lunch meats and bacon. Buy only lean cuts of meat; trim off all external fat.

WHERE'S THE BEEF?

If you have been avoiding red meat because of its fat content, take heart. The beef industry is trying some innovative techniques for producing leaner cuts. Ranchers are trimming the fat from beef by cross-breeding their stock with cattle that are naturally lean. Some ranchers are importing European breeds like the Chianina from Italy and Limousin from France. Other ranchers are leaving their cattle in the feedlots for shorter periods of time— 100 to 110 days instead of the traditional 120 days.

Not only are ranchers trying to bring beef back to the dinner table of health-conscious Americans, butchers at packing houses and supermarkets are also trimming the fat. Instead of the customary 1/2 inch or more of external fat, they are trimming the fat around the edge of the meat to about 1/4 inch.

The United States Department of Agriculture (USDA) has proposed that beef labeled "lean" or "low-fat" cannot contain more than 10 percent fat by weight and that "extra-lean" meat be limited to 5 percent fat. "Leaner" or "light" meat would have at least 25 percent less fat than regular cuts, or have less than 10 percent fat. The USDA is also proposing to change the name of "good" grade meat to "select." Good grade meat is lower in fat than choice or prime grades. The term "natural" simply means that a product is minimally processed and contains no artificial ingredients. It does not mean that a meat is free of antibodies or hormones.

The meat recipes in this book keep fat to a minimum by: (1) using lean cuts— 10 percent or less fat and (2) trimming external fat very close before cooking. Other ways that fat is kept to a minimum is by using smaller quantities of meat in stir-fry dishes, in pilafs or combined with pasta or vegetables.

POULTRY

Americans are eating less beef—15 pounds less per year, and more poultry than 10 years ago. Nutritionally, poultry has about the same amount of calories, protein and cholesterol as lean red meat. The difference is that poultry contains less saturated fat. Twenty-five percent of the fat in poultry is saturated as opposed to 35 to 45 percent in beef. Poultry also contains less vitamin B_{12} and zinc than red meat.

The way poultry is prepared influences its saturated fat. To keep it low, bake, broil, or grill poultry and take off the skin before eating. Limit the sauces and condiments served with poultry. One-fourth cup of hollandaise sauce adds about 20 grams of saturated fat.

THE FISH STORY

Fish has always been a good low-calorie, low-cholesterol food choice. Recent studies are suggesting that the Omega-3-fatty acids found in fish are more effective in fighting blood cholesterol than the fatty acids found in vegetable oils.

COMPARISON OF LEAN MEAT & POULTRY PRODUCTS

MEAT 3 oz. cooked	CAL	FAT % by wt.	FAT % of cal.	FAT % of sat.	CHOL (mg)	PRO %USRDA	IRON %USRDA
Sirloin tip roast, "good" grade, trimmable fat removed	156	6.7	33	37	69	38	14
Top loin steak, "good" grade, trimmable fat removed	163	7.5	36	40	65	38	12
Hamburger meat (not graded by USDA)	240	17.6	57	39	87	37	12
Lamb chop, loin cut*	184	9.7	41	50	81	40	10
Leg of lamb, sirloin*	175	9.2	41	50	79	38	10
Veal chop, loin cut*	192	9.0	36	+	135	44	9
Veal cutlet, round cut*	150	7.2	37	+	112	34	9
Chicken breast, without skin	131	4.1	24	27	64	36	5
Ham	191	6.4	26	+	+	51	11
Pork tenderloin	142	4.8	26	35	78	38	4

*Values are approximate. USDA is currently gathering data on lamb and veal for a special nutrition handbook.   +Figures not available.
Tufts University Diet & Nutrition Letter. Vol. 5, No. 10. December, 1987.

Generally speaking, you should eat at least 7 ounces of fish a week.

To keep fish low in fat, you must prepare it correctly. Breading, frying, adding a cream sauce or wrapping it in puff pastry will boost its fat content substantially. Bake, grill, broil or microwave your fish for the most nutritional benefit. Try the Fish Fillets with Green Peppers (page 116) or Deviled Fish Kabobs (page 112) for two delicious ways to include more fish in your diet.

HOW TO CHOOSE AN EXERCISE PROGRAM THAT IS RIGHT FOR YOU

Eating the right foods is important, but it is only one side of the fitness coin.

Exercise is also important for looking and feeling your best. A regular exercise program will help you:
- Increase blood circulation
- Increase muscle tone
- Burn more calories
- Decrease blood cholesterol
- Reduce tension

When the going gets tough, the tough get—injured. Contrary to popular belief, the old adage of "no pain, no gain" simply is not true. An exercise program does not have to be painful in order to enhance your health and improve your appearance.

What should you look for in an exercise program and how should you get started?

To choose an activity that is right for

you, decide why you want to start exercising. Do you want to make your heart stronger in order to decrease your chances of heart attack? Do you want to increase your endurance in order to ski longer and harder than last year? Do you want to increase your strength in order to become a better wind-surfer? Or do you simply want to, lose weight and tone your muscles in order to feel and look your best?

If general conditioning—improved endurance and greater muscle tone—is your objective, there are some principles to keep in mind before starting an exercise program.

TIPS FOR GENERAL CONDITIONING

In order to improve your conditioning—to exert more energy for a longer period of time with less effort—you must engage in some kind of "aerobic" activity. When you are out of shape, you huff and puff walking uphill because your body is starved for oxygen. Aerobic exercise helps your heart and other muscles use oxygen more efficiently. Aerobics also helps your muscles develop more of the enzymes they need to burn fat. Examples of aerobic exercise include walking, bicycling, jogging, swimming, aerobic dance or using exercise equipment such as a rowing machine or a cross-country ski machine. Research suggests that aerobic exercise is most effective if done continuously for 20 to 40 minutes, 3 to 4 times a week.

Your heart rate during exercise is the best way to determine if you are getting the most benefit from your workout. Sixty to seventy percent of your maximum heart rate—called your target heart rate (THR)—is considered the most effective training pulse for maximum cardiovascular and fat burning benefits.

Finding Your Pulse

You can find your pulse either on the thumb side of your wrist (palm up) or in the groove on your neck. To find your resting heart rate (RHR), take your pulse for a full minute when you first wake up, still lying down, on two consecutive mornings. Then average the two numbers. Your resting heart rate becomes lower as you become more conditioned.

Finding Your Pulse While Exercising

To check your heart rate during exercise, stop about 5 minutes into your exercise and place the fingers (not thumb) of one hand on the thumbside of your wrist of the other hand. Press firmly, then gradually let up until you feel a pulse. Count your pulse for 6 seconds using the minute hand of a watch. Add a zero to the number of beats you count to determine your exercising heart rate per minute. Compare your exercising heart rate to your estimated target rate and make any necessary adjustments. For example, if your exercising heart rate is higher than your target rate, slow down. If it is lower, increase the intensity of your exercise. The important thing is to keep moving. Many researchers support the theory that the number of times you exercise each week or the number of times your heart beats during exercise is not as important as simply moving your body more—becoming more physically active during the day. For instance, use the stairs instead of the elevator. When you go to the store, park further from the door than you usually do and walk a few extra yards. Walk around the park after dinner instead of walking to the television.

The person in the box opposite should be exercising at about 141 beats per minute for at least 20 minutes for maximum aerobic benefit. The most important thing to remember when you exercise is to listen to your body—the opposite equation is simply a guideline. Tune into your body for specific signals if an exercise program is too intense or not intense enough. Some people can reach their target rate with a brisk walk, others have to run 7-minute miles in order to get their heart pumping hard enough to reach 60 to 70 percent of their maximum heart rate.

Aerobic exercise is not only good for conditioning your heart and lungs, but it draws upon fat stores for energy. Thus a longer, less-intense activity is more effective in reducing your percent body fat than a short, intense activity. In other words a 30 minute walk is better for you than running at a quick clip for 15 minutes.

The key to making exercise a habit is to find an activity that you enjoy. Whether it is swimming, bicycling or walking

HOW TO DETERMINE YOUR TARGET HEART RATE

Target Heart Rates

    220

    -Your age
_____

    (maximum heart rate)

    -Your resting heart rate
_____

_____ x 60% for begin
ning exercisers or

_____ x 70% for mod
erate exercisers or

_____ x 80% for competi
tive athletes
_____

    + **Resting heart rate**
_____

    (target heart rate)

For example, if you are 35 years old, just beginning an exercise program, have a resting heart rate of 75 beats per minute, your calculations would be as follows:

    220

    - 35 (age)
_____

    185

    - 75 (RHR)
_____

    110

    x .60 (fitness level)
_____

    66

    + 75 (RHR)
_____

    141 target heart rate

around your block, just make sure your heart rate is elevated and beating close to your target level.

The type of activity you do is not important. If you get bored with one exercise—mix it up. Bicycle on one day, take an aerobics class the next. Many of my patients are amazed that they can lose inches and body fat by walking briskly for 30 to 40 minutes a day. The specific exercise is not as important as taking 30 minutes of your day to be physically active.

Toning Muscles

Muscles stay toned according to the use and disuse principle—the more the muscle is used, the stronger and more firm it becomes. Any kind of resistance training such as lifting free weights, using weight machines or using hand-held weights will increase toning. The important thing is consistency—to include some kind of resistance training 2 to 3 times a week. As the exercise becomes easier, you can gradually increase the weight for greater strength-gain.

Exercises which use the body for resistance also improve muscle tone. Bent-knee sit-ups, push-ups, leg lifts and arm lifts are all good toning exercises.

HEART RATES		
AGE	MAX. HEART RATE	70%
20-29	200-191	140-134
30-39	190-181	133-137
40-49	180-171	126-120
50-59	170-161	119-113
60-69	160-151	112-106

CHOOSING THE RIGHT EXERCISE FOR YOU

For general conditioning and increased muscle tone, a combination of aerobic activity and resistance training is most effective. Some suggestions for combined exercises include activities such as:

• Riding a stationary bicycle that has moveable handlebars to create a rowing-type movement.

• Using a rowing machine.

• Using a cross-country ski machine.

• Walking or jogging while carrying hand-weights.

• Participating in an exercise class that includes bent-knee sit-ups, push-ups, leg lifts or other resistance exercises, with or without hand-held weights.

• Swimming or bicycling 3 times a week and lifting weight 2 times a week.

GETTING STARTED

To help you get started, take your calendar or appointment book and actually block out at least 20 minutes in next week's schedule to walk around a nearby park. Continue to schedule time until you are in a routine of exercising at least 20 minutes 3 to 4 times a week.

Sign a contract with an exercise partner for support and motivation in sticking with a program. Determine the time and place ahead of time and don't let your partner down. You are not committing yourself to one place or one activity, but to a process to raise, sustain and lower your pulse through whichever activity you choose.

Use time as your exercise guide at first. For instance, simply plan to move continuously for 30 minutes, then gradually add other factors such as increasing the intensity of your exercise or carrying weights while you exercise.

If playing a competitive game is more your style, you might consider a non-stop game of racquetball or handball. Remember that your heart rate should stay elevated at 60 to 70 percent of your maximum heart rate for about 30 minutes in order to derive the maximum benefits from your exercise. An aerobic program will include all of the following components:

Warm-Up (5 minutes)

The warm-up is to limber muscles and gradually ease into an activity at a slow, easy pace. It prepares muscles and joints for exercise and helps prevent injuries. Allow at least a 5 minute warm-up.

Aerobic Component (20 minutes)

The aerobic portion of your exercise program can be any vigorous movement that involves the large muscle groups of your body. Keep in mind the 3 FIT factors of aerobic exercise:

• FREQUENCY: 3 to 5 times per week.

• INTENSITY: Exercise vigorously enough to elevate your heart rate to 60 to 70 percent of its maximum capacity. If you can't talk comfortably while you are exercising, you are probably exercising too hard. If you can sing while you workout, you're not working hard enough.

• TIME: Maintain your target heart rate for at least 20 minutes. To prevent injuries and increase variety, switch between impact exercises like aerobic dance and running and non-impact activities like bicycling or swimming. The aerobic segment should last at least 20 minutes.

Cool-Down (5 minutes)

The purpose of the cool-down is to ease out of your activity slowly, and to prevent injuries from stiff muscles. After at least 20 minutes of aerobic exercise, slow your pace gradually until your heart rate returns to normal. The more fit you are, the quicker you recover. After walking slowly for 3 to 5 minutes your pulse should be below 100 beats per minute. After your heart rate has returned to normal gradually stretch your muscles while they are warm to prevent stiffness later. A cool-down should last at least 5 minutes.

Keep a record of how much you exercise each day. An exercise log provides a sense of accomplishment and motivation to stick with your exercise program. It is also a great way to get to know your body better and to determine which exercises are best for you. Record the date, the type of activity and the length of time you exercised at your target heart rate.

Whatever type of exercise you choose to do, remember to do the following suggestions:

• Learn to take your pulse and use

your target heart rate while you exercise.

- Alternate impact and nonimpact exercises to prevent injury and add variety to your workouts.
- Set realistic fitness goals.
- Set a regular schedule of exercise throughout the week—don't just exercise on the weekends.
- Exercise in the proper shoes, clothing, and with the proper equipment.
- If you participate in an impact exercise, make sure the surface is safe for the specific activity. For example the floor for an aerobic dance class should be spring or coil based under wood—not concrete. If you jog or walk, a surface that gives is best such as asphalt, grass, or soft dirt.
- Listen to your body and remember—no pain, no injuries.

EXERCISING AT HOME: VIDEOS

Hectic schedules demand handy workouts you can do right at home. Home videos can make exercising both convenient and inexpensive. Since alternating workouts is the key to avoiding injury and preventing boredom, exchange exercise tapes with a friend or have a few different tapes on hand to add variety.

The problem with exercising at home is that in the privacy of your own home, there is no instructor to supervise your moves and make sure you are doing the exercises correctly. Some specific guidelines to keep in mind when looking for a safe exercise video include the following suggestions:

- Consult your physician before starting an exercise program, especially if you are over age 35 and out of shape.
- Select a tape that matches your fitness level. If you have been working out regularly for the last year, a beginner's tape is not for you.
- Make sure you warm up for 5 minutes and cool down for at least 5 minutes. If a video routine does not contain these components, add them yourself.
- Monitor your heart rate while you are exercising. You should work within your target level for 20 to 30 minutes.
- Limit your workouts to 20 to 30 minutes, 3 to 5 times a week. Exercising more than 5 times a week can lead to injury and fatigue.

- Listen to your body and take precautions to protect your back and joints. Use an exercise mat if you need it, and avoid using weights that are too heavy.
- Pay close attention to the video instructor and concentrate on each specific exercise.
- Align yourself properly to the TV screen. Standing directly in front of the screen is best.

The following videos are recommended when evaluated for safety, leader qualities, visual/audio qualities, music and equipment: (information adapted from "Exercise on the Home Front" by Wayne Osness, PhD., SHAPE Magazine, May 1987.)
AEROBIC VIDEOS:
Kathy Smith's Ultimate Video Workout
STRENGTHENING:
Body Band Workout with Tamilee Webb
LOW-IMPACT VIDEOS:
No-Jump Aerobics with Charlene Pickett
BODY CONTOURING:
Esquire's Great Body Total Body Tone Up with Deborah Crocker
STRETCHING/FLEXIBILITY:
Doreen Rivers Presents Stretch for Life
PREGNANCY:
JACOG Pregnancy Exercise Program

EXERCISING AT HOME: EQUIPMENT

Exercise equipment such as a rowing machine, a stationary bicycle, a cross-country ski machine or a weight machine lets you bike, row, lift weights and ski without leaving your living room. Last year Americans spent over one million dollars on equipment to use at home. Keep in mind the following suggestions before jumping on the at-home exercise band wagon:

Try out the equipment before you buy. Make sure it fits your specific fitness goals, time constraints and financial abilities. The stationary bicycle, the rowing machine and the cross-country ski machine are three of the best pieces of conditioning equipment available.

A combination of aerobic exercise and resistance training is an ideal way to increase endurance, improve conditioning and tone your muscles.

Strengthening Your Muscles

If your exercise goal is primarily to

• Resistance should be controllable and numbered.

• Seat and handlebars should be comfortable and adjustable.

• Pedals should spin easily. Straps that hold your feet in place are a good idea to have.

ROWING MACHINE

• The best types have a heavy duty steel frame.

• Prices vary greatly, but a good machine will cost $300 to $400.

• Look for a comfortable seat that slides easily.

• The resistance device should be adjustable and produce smooth movements.

• You should be able to straighten your legs when working out.

• Pivoting footrests are more desirable than fixed ones.

CROSS-COUNTRY SKI MACHINE

• A good machine will cost about $500.

• Look for sturdy construction and smooth action.

• A machine should stimulate the actual motion of cross-country skiing.

WEIGHT MACHINE

Weight training includes hand weights, free weights (barbells) or weight machines. Weight machines are safer than free weights, but are very expensive ($1800 to $4500). Keep in mind the following suggestions before purchasing any type of weight machine:

• Look for a sturdy steel frame that is well-padded at the contact points.

• Cables should be made of heavy steel. Avoid plastic pulleys.

• Make sure the weight increments are right for your level of fitness.

Keep in mind the same principles of warming up, maintaining your target heart rate and cooling down when using home exercise equipment.

EXERCISING WITH A GROUP

A conditioning or toning class at your local health club is another way to increase endurance and tone your muscles. Make sure the teacher is certified by a reputable organization such as The American College of Sports Medicine (ACSM), The Aerobics and Fitness Association of America (AFAA) or the International Dance-Exercise Association (IDEA). The instructor should allow time to warm up and cool down, and should allow you to work at your own pace. Other criteria to use when looking for an exercise class include factors such as:

Instructor Evaluation

• Has the instructor had any training in anatomy, physiology, kinesiology or prevention of injuries?

• Is the instructor certified in cardiopulmonary resuscitation (CPR)?

• Does the instructor explain specific exercises and how to do them in a controlled manner?

• Does the instructor establish eye contact and periodically move around the room to help participants with specific movements?

• Does the instructor allow time for and explain how to take heart rates during the aerobics portion of class?

• Does the class seem to move smoothly from one exercise to the next?

• Does the instructor stay after class to answer questions?

Class Evaluation

• Is the warm-up at least 5 minutes long?

• Does the warm-up prepare you for the moves you will be doing in the aerobic segment of class?

• Do the aerobic exercises gradually increase in intensity beginning slowly so your heart rate slowly reaches your target level?

• Is the aerobic segment 20 to 30 minutes in length?

• Do you cool down gradually for 4 to 5 minutes—moving your legs until your heart rate slows to 120 beats per minute before you begin the calisthenic portion of class?

• Does the instructor explain how to perform each calisthenic exercise correctly and explain which muscle group you are using?

• Are the calisthenics varied so that you don't overfatigue any one muscle group? Are you working opposing muscle groups to promote muscular balance?

• Does the final cool-down last at least 8 to 10 minutes and incorporate static stretches of the muscle groups used during the aerobic portion of class?

- Are you instructed to hold your stretches for 20 to 30 seconds?
- Does the instructor remain after class to answer questions?

War on Fat

Resistance training is great for toning muscles, but it has very little affect on the fat that lays beneath the muscle. The only way to get rid of this fat is to do some type of aerobic activity that boosts your heart rate to your target level for 30 to 40 minutes. Any exercise or machine that actually moves your body for you without raising your pulse does nothing to burn your fat stores. You may tone your muscles, but the fat is still there.

A combination of aerobic exercise and resistance training is an ideal way to increase endurance, improve conditioning and tone your muscles.

Strengthening Your Muscles

If your exercise goal is primarily to increase your strength, specific resistance training is for you. A structured schedule that specifies the amount of weight and number of repetitions for each exercise is necessary to increase muscular strength. Generally speaking, fewer repetitions with a heavier weight will increase strength, while more repetitions with a lighter weight will increase endurance. The interval of rest between repetitions also plays a role in strength training. For assistance in developing a strength training program that is specific for you, consult the exercise physiologist or trainer at your health club or sports medicine clinic.

FINAL WORD

There is no time like the present to start exercising. If you already participate in a regular program—keep up the good work. If you are a compulsive exerciser—be kind to your body, listen to what it is telling you. Skip working out one to two days a week. You'll be amazed how much more energy you have, and how much healthier you will feel.

SPECIAL NUTRITIONAL NEEDS FOR ATHLETES

Besides more energy, an active person needs more B vitamins and fluids than a sedentary person. The B vitamins can be easily provided by the extra calories that an athlete eats. Fluids, however, are a different story.

FLUIDS

Fluid replacement is crucial for all active people. Adequate fluids are important for blood circulation, urine production and body temperature control. Unfortunately, the body's thirst mechanism is not a very reliable indicator of when a person needs something to drink. This mechanism is triggered only after fluid losses reach 1 percent of a person's total body weight. For instance, if you weigh 150 pounds, you wouldn't actually feel thirsty until you lost about 1-1/2 pounds in sweat. Your physical performance will decline after losing 2 to 3 percent of your total body weight. A 7 to 10 percent loss of weight can result in heat stroke, and in extreme cases, death.

An athlete can theoretically lose 14 pounds of sweat over a 4-hour competition unless fluids are ingested during the event. Ultra-endurance athletes who exercise at least 4 hours are not the only ones at risk of dehydration. Runners in races as short as 1OK have reported feeling disoriented and incoherant due to heat, humidity and insufficient fluid intake.

Fluid replacement is important before, during and after an athletic event. The following suggestions will help assure that you are well-hydrated:

- Drink at least 8 (8-ounce) glasses of fluid a day—any food or beverage counts. For example, water, lemonade, juice, watermelon, oranges and lettuce all contribute a substantial amount of fluid to your diet.
- Drink before you feel thirsty. Remember that your thirst mechanism is delayed. You actually need fluids before you feel thirsty.
- During hot weather, drink 8 to 10 ounces of cold water every 20 minutes while exercising.
- During the day of competition, drink up to two hours before the event. Drink a glass of water about 5 minutes before competition begins if possible.
- To replace body fluids after exercising, drink 2 cups of water for every

pound lost while exercising (Weigh before and after exercising to determine this). For example, if you lose 4 pounds during an event, you need to drink the equivalent of 8 (8-ounce) glasses of fluid. Continue to drink fluids for a few hours after exercise—until your pre-exercise weight is regained.

How to Prevent Overheating

Exercise increases body temperature, and sweating is the body's way of cooling itself. The more you exercise, the more water you lose through sweat. For your body to cool properly, the sweat must be able to evaporate. Excessive layers of clothing and high humidity prevent this evaporation and you can become overheated.

The following suggestions can prevent overheating during exercise:

• When training or competing in hot weather, drink 8 to 10 ounces of fluid every 20 minutes. NEVER restrict fluids during exercise.

• If the type of exercise allows, carry a water bottle with you. If you can't carry water with you, plan to take frequent water breaks, and train in areas where water is readily available.

• Be extra cautious if you train in high humidity. Plan to train early in the morning or after 4:00 p.m. to avoid the compounded effects of high temperatures and high humidity.

• Wear loose-fitting, light-colored clothing. Never wear rubberized clothing for any reason.

• Wait until you are completely recovered from exercising before taking a shower, sauna, whirlpool or bath. Your blood vessels are already dilated because of the heat generated through exercise. Sitting in hot water or a sauna opens the blood vessels even more. More blood is diverted through these dilated vessels, resulting in less blood going to the brain. This reduced blood flow to the brain can result in drowsiness or even unconsciousness—a very dangerous situation if you are in or around hot water or high heat.

• Be aware of the early signs of overheating. These include: "goose bumps," chilling, throbbing, pressure in the head, unsteadiness, nausea and dry skin.

QUESTIONS & ANSWERS

Q: What is the best thing to drink before, during and after exercise?

A: Plain water is the best fluid replacement. Cold water is absorbed faster than warm. Plain water is absorbed faster than drinks that contain sugar such as juice, soft drinks, or sports beverages.

Q: I hear a lot about electrolytes when referring to fluid replacement. What are they?

A: Electrolytes are "charged" particles that play an essential part in the chemical reactions that occur in your cells during exercise. When a person sweats, not only is water lost, but the balance of important electrolytes such as sodium and potassium is upset. When this balance is upset, physical performance declines. Drinking plenty of water is one way to prevent the loss of important electrolytes. Other factors that can throw your electrolytes off balance include vomitting, diarrhea, diuretics and excessive salt intake.

Q: Are commercial sports drinks a good way to replace electrolytes?

A: Most electrolyte drinks are more expensive and actually contain fewer electrolytes than other beverages. For example, 8 ounces of orange juice contains 25 times more potassium than the same amount of Gatorade.

To make your own electrolyte replacement drink, combine:
    4 cups water
    1/4 cup frozen orange juice
        concentrate
    2/3 teaspoon salt
    Chill thoroughly before drinking.
Some endurance athletes prefer "flat" soft drinks or diluted juice to help replace electrolytes and glycogen. To dilute fruit juice, add one-half the amount of water to the regular strength juice. To make a soft drink "flat," open and leave it in the refrigerator overnight.

Q: Isn't drinking beer after an endurance race a food way to replace depleted glycogen?

A: Despite popular belief, beer contributes very little carbohydrate to the diet. Most of the calories come from the alcohol. Alcohol has a diuretic effect on the body. Rather than quench your thirst, alcohol will cause you to lose water and become more thirsty.

Q: I perspire a lot. Shouldn't I take salt tablets?

A: No. A well-conditioned athlete loses very little sodium through sweat. When an athlete perspires, vital body fluid is lost, and the salt around the cells becomes more concentrated. Taking salt tablets increases the salt concentration even more and is strongly discouraged in most athletic situations. Instead of salt tablets, you should drink plenty of water and add a little extra salt to your food.

Q: How do I replace the potassium I lose through sweat?

A: We do not know exactly how much potassium is lost through sweat, but it is probably not enough to affect physical performance. Most nutritionists recommend replacing the potassium lost through sweat by eating plenty of fresh fruits and vegetables. See below for the potassium content of some common foods.

VITAMINS & MINERALS

Q: I have heard vitamins and minerals do not contribute any energy to my diet—what do they do?

A: Vitamins and minerals are like a choreographer in a musical play. They tell the body what chemical reactions to perform to produce energy without actually providing the energy for the reactions themselves. They are catalysts that enable the body to function properly.

Q: As an athlete, what extra vitamins and minerals do I need—and where should I get them?

A: Most nutritionists agree that an active person does not need excessive amounts of any vitamin or mineral. Eating a variety of lightly processed foods is the best way to fulfill your nutritional requirements. Supplements are for people with special nutritional needs, or for someone who is unable to eat a balanced diet.

Q: How can I be sure I am eating a balanced diet, and that the foods I do eat contain the nutrients that they should.

A: The basic 2-2-4-4 eating plan—2 servings of milk, 2 (3-ounce) servings of meat, 4 servings of breads and cereals and 4 servings of fruits and vegetables—provide more than enough of the vitamins and minerals that you need. Even if the nutri-

POTASSIUM CONTENT OF COMMON FOODS

FOOD	POTASSIUM (mg.)	CALORIES
Baked potato without skin (1 medium-size)	503	95
Beans, baked in tomato sauce (1/2 cup)	304	128
Raisins (1/2 cup)	601	240
Banana (1 medium-size)	451	105
Avocado (1/4)	274	76
Orange (1 medium-size)	250	65
Orange juice, frozen concentrate, diluted (8 ounces)	474	112
Tomato juice, canned (8 ounces)	598	41
Gatorade (8 ounces)	23	39
Milk, skim (8 ounces)	406	86
Broccoli, cooked (1 stalk)	267	32
Spinach, cooked (1/2 cup)	291	21
Beef, chuck, cooked (3 ounces)	333	294
Poultry, chicken—white meat without skin (3 ounces)	212	138
Fish, flounder, baked (3 ounces)	304	128

The average person should consume at least 3000 mg of potassium a day. An athlete who trains in hot weather or who tries to supersaturate his muscles with glycogen needs 300 to 800 mg more potassium a day.

Adapted from Pennington, Jean, and Church, Helen. *Food Values of Portions Commonly Used.* 14th Edition, Harper & Row: New York. 1985.

tional quality of your food is poor, the chances of you not getting enough of a specific vitamin or mineral is highly unlikely. Developing a vitamin deficiency is even more doubtful.

CALCIUM

Q: With all the emphasis on osteoporosis, shouldn't I be concerned about getting enough calcium?

A: Osteoporosis is a condition characterized by weak brittle bones. Low calcium intake is associated with this condition. An adult needs at least 800 to 1000 milligrams of calcium a day, or the equivalent of 2 to 3 glasses of milk. If you do not drink milk, consider the following suggestions for increasing your calcium intake:

- Select hard cheeses like Swiss and Gruyère. They have more calcium than soft cheeses, such as cream cheese or Brie, and cheese-food products.
- Add grated Parmesan and Romano cheese to casseroles, salads and sandwich fillings.

- Use part-skim ricotta instead of cottage cheese for an extra 259 mg of calcium per 1/2 cup.
- Select dairy products that are fortified with nonfat dry milk solids.
- Use canned salmon with bones for sandwich fillings, casseroles or salads.
- Be choosy if you use green leafy vegetables as a calcium source. Spinach and Swiss chard contain oxalates which prevent the body from absorbing the calcium. Eat collard greens, turnip greens or broccoli instead.
- Buy tofu that is processed with calcium. It has about 130 mg of calcium per 3-1/2-ounce serving.
- Popular Mexican foods contribute a substantial amount of calcium to the diet. A cheese enchilada made with a corn tortilla and 1/4 cup of grated cheese provides about 250 mg of calcium.

Q: If I decide to take a calcium supplement, which kind is the best?

A: Calcium carbonate is a popular supplement because it contains more calcium per

APPROXIMATE CALCIUM CONTENT OF COMMON FOODS

FOOD GROUP	AMOUNT OF CALCIUM (mg.)
DAIRY	
Plain yogurt (8 ounces)	400
Non-fat dry milk powder (1/2 cup)	400
Skim, low-fat, or buttermilk (1 cup)	300
Fruit-flavored yogurt (8 ounces)	300
Ricotta cheese, part-skim (1/2 cup)	300
Parmesan, Romano, Swiss cheese (1 ounce)	300
Cheddar, Jack, Muenster cheese (1 ounce)	200
American cheese (1 ounce)	150
Ice Cream, Ice milk (1/2 cup)	150
Camembert cheese (1 ounce)	100
Cottage cheese (1/2 cup)	50
BREADS & CEREALS	
Pancake (1 (6-inch))	150
Bread (2 slices)	50
Corn tortilla, (1 (6-inch))	50
FRUIT	
Orange (1 medium-size)	50
Figs (2)	50
PROTEIN FOODS	
Canned sardines with the bone (3 ounces)	400
Sockeye salmon, canned with bone (3 ounces)	300
Tofu (4 ounces)	150

Adapted from Pennington, Jean, and Church, Helen. *Food Values of Portions Commonly Used.* 14th Edition, Harper & Row: New York. 1985.

tablet, is easier to absorb, is inexpensive and is readily available in the form of antacids like Tums or in the form of ground oyster shell.

IRON:

Q: What is "sports anemia"?

A: Sports anemia occurs when your body's iron stores become low or depleted. It is fairly common among endurance athletes. To decrease your risk of developing this condition, consider the following suggestions:

• Monitor your weight before and after exercising. For every 8 pounds of weight lost through sweat, you can lose up to 1 mg of iron. Make a special effort to replace this iron on a daily basis.

• Combine and prepare foods in a way that enhances iron absorption (see next answer).

• Consume enough calories to assure an adequate iron intake. If your food does not supply enough iron, take a supplement. The following chart lists the iron content of some common foods.

Q: I have heard that iron is important for energy. How can I be sure I am getting enough iron in my diet?

A: Iron plays an important role both in transporting oxygen to the muscles and producing energy within the muscle. Men need about 10 milligrams a day, while women need 18 milligrams.

You absorb only about 10 percent of the iron contained in the food you eat. If you limit your calories or don't eat red meat, you should probably take an iron supplement. To enhance the amount of iron you absorb from your food, try the following suggestions:

• Eat a food high in vitamin C along with a food high in iron. For example, eat an iron-fortified cereal along with a glass of orange juice.

• Limit the amount of coffee and tea you drink with meals. Substances called tannins in both beverages inhibit the absorption of iron.

• Eat red meat with vegetables that are rich in iron at the same meal for greater iron absorption.

• Include moderate amounts of red meat in your diet. Three ounces of poultry provides only 1 mg of iron, while 3 ounces of beef contains about 4 mg.

• If you choose to limit red meat, eat plenty of enriched or fortified grain products. Tofu and cooked dried beans are good sources of iron; be sure to combine them with a whole-grain food to make a complete protein.

• Check the labels on the bread products that you buy to ensure that they are made with enriched flour. Many products labeled "natural" contain unenriched flour which is lower in iron.

• Cook acidic foods, like tomato

IRON CONTENT OF COMMON FOODS

FOOD ITEM	IRON (mg.)	CALORIES
Iron fortified cereal, 3/4 cup	18.0	108
Bran Flakes cereal with raisins, 3/4 cup	13.0	108
Liver, beef, cooked, 3 oz.	12.1	222
Liver, calf, cooked, 3 oz.	7.5	195
Prune juice, 4 oz.	5.0	98
Beef, cooked, 3 oz.	3.1	212
Baked beans, 1/2 cup	2.6	153
Raisins, 1/2 cup	2.5	210
Kidney beans, canned, 1/2 cup	2.3	115
Tofu, 2-1/2" x 2-1/2" x 1" piece	2.3	86
Pork, cooked, 3 oz.	2.2	246

Adapted from Pennington, Jean, and Church, Helen. *Food Values of Portions Commonly Used.* 14th Edition, Harper & Row: New York. 1985.

CAFFEINE CONTENT OF COMMON FOODS

	CAFFEINE CONTENT (mg)
Coffee per cup:	
Instant	61-70
Percolated	97-125
Dripolated	137-153
Tea per cup:	
Weak	18-45
Strong	70-90
Instant tea-hot	55
Instant ice tea	72
Cocoa (Dutch) per cup	10-17
Chocolate candy bar (1 oz.)	25
Cola beverage (12 oz.)	32-65
Coca-Cola	65
Dr. Pepper	61
Mountain Dew	55
Diet Dr. Pepper	54
Tab	49
Pepsi-Cola	43
RC Cola	34
Diet RC	33
Diet-Rite	32
5-grain aspirin tablet	15-30
"Stay awake" tablet	110

Reprinted from *Nutrition Action Healthletter*, which is available from the center for Science in the Public Interest, 1501 16th Street, NW, Washington, D.C. 20036, for $19.95 for 10 issues. Copyright 1988.

sauce, in cast-iron skillets. Some of the iron from the skillet actually leaches out into the sauce.

• Use meat bones when making soup stock. Boiling the bones can increase the iron content of the broth.

Q: Besides calcium and iron, are there any other vitamins and minerals that are important for physical activity?

A: The B vitamins, vitamin C, potassium and magnesium are all important for muscular contraction. Your needs for these nutrients are easily met through a balanced diet.

ENHANCING PHYSICAL PERFORMANCE

An athlete is always looking for that competitive edge—that little something that will push him closer to realizing his full potential. New products appear on the market daily that promise strength and stamina. Today it is amino acid supplementation, CoEnzyme Q or bee pollen. Tomorrow it will be something else. Until an energy enhancing product has stood the test of time, nutritionists will continue to recommend a balanced diet, plenty of fluids, hard work and good genes as the best way to enhance your performance.

CAFFEINE

Q: I have heard that caffeine will improve my endurance. Is this true?

A: Research shows that caffeine stimulates the release of fat into the blood. Since your muscles prefer to burn fat for endurance activity, drinking a caffeinated beverage before exercising would spare your glycogen stores. Theoretically, you could exercise longer before reaching exhaustion. Two to three cups of coffee (or about 280 mg of caffeine) one hour before an endurance event seems to do the trick. Experiment to see what works best for you.

STEROIDS

Q: I lift weights at a local gym and keep hearing about steroids. What are they and what do they do?

A: Anabolic steroids are a synthetic derivative of the male hormone testosterone. The use of anabolic steroids in athletics has a colorful history dating back to the 1960s when champion wrestlers gobbled them like candy in hopes of "bulking up" and increasing muscle strength. Today they are popular among athletes in sports such as football, wrestling and power-lifting. While many athletes—both male and female, believe that steroids improve their performance, the health hazards are an important consideration for anyone who entertains the idea of taking them. The negative side-effects of steroids include:

• Increased risk of heart disease. The more steroids you take, the more likely you are to have a heart attack.

• Increased chance of serious liver disorders.

• Hormonal imbalances in both men and women. Women become more like men and men become more like women.

• Water retention. Steroids can cause a 30 pound weight gain in 30 days. Excessive water can interfere with the electrolyte balance within the cell.

CARBOHYDRATE LOADING

Q: I compete in 5 and lOK fun runs and hear a lot about carbohydrate loading. What is it, and can it improve my performance?

A: Carbohydrate loading is a diet and exercise regime that seems to enhance endurance. It is most effective for events that last over 45 minutes.

Research shows that muscles can actually store more glycogen—more energy, if they are completely depleted and then "reloaded." This deplete and load regime causes the muscles to becomes super-saturated with glycogen.

Traditionally, carbohydrate loading was initiated 5 to 6 days before an endurance event. The first 3 days—the depletion phase, consisted of strenuous workouts and a low carbohydrate diet. The loading phase—the last 3 days, is a time for light exercise and a high carbohydrate diet. Many endurance athletes prefer to omit the depletion phase because of the strain it has on the heart and kidneys, and because of the extreme fatigue experienced during that time. Instead, they lighten up on training and load up on carbohydrates 2 to 3 days before their event.

Q: What are some ideas for high carbohydrate meals that I can eat 2 to 3 days before my triathalon competition?

A: The recipes in this book offer many mouth-watering possibilities. Some sample menus are included below:

    Spaghetti with Marinara Sauce
       (page 138)
    French bread
    Green beans
    Apple Strudel (page 183)
    Ice water or fruit juice
         -or-
    Ricotta Cheese Pancakes with
       Strawberries (page 189)
    Canadian bacon slice
    Fruit juice
         -or-
    Stuffed baked potato filled with
       turkey and steamed broccoli
    Cranberry Orange Bread (page 172)
    Fruit salad
    Ice water
         -or-
    Lamb Pilaf (page 90)
    No-Knead Dilly Bread (page 165)
    Sliced tomatoes
    Spicy Poached Pears (page 178)

EATING BEFORE, DURING & AFTER COMPETING

Q: Besides high carbohydrate foods, what else should I eat before competing?

A: Whether you run lOK races, play competitive tennis or play recreational softball, there are certain principles to keep in mind for your pregame meal:

• Go heavy on the carbohydrates since they are easier to digest. Cereal with fruit, a lean meat sandwich, yogurt or noodle soup are all good choices before you exercise.

• Go light on high-fat foods like bacon, steak, butter, margarine, salad dressing and mayonnaise. They take longer to leave your stomach.

• Eat about 2 hours before exercising. If you are nervous, allow more time so your food will be completely digested. Include plenty of fluids such as water, juice or weak tea.

Q: Should I worry about eating something while I am competing?

A: Unless you are an ultra-endurance athlete and exercising for 4 hours or more, eating during an event is probably not necessary. Some popular foods among triathletes and ultra-marathoners are things like mashed banana, figs, bread, cookies, oranges and applesauce. Commercially prepared drinks like "Exceed" are also available to replace fluids and provide easily digestable carbohydrate.

Q: After competing, I am ready to sink my teeth into something besides bread and pasta, what would you suggest?

A: Two important objectives of a post-game meal include replenishing glycogen stores and replacing lost fluid. Some ideas for eating after competing include:

Fisherman's Spaghetti (page 124)
Grilled Garlic bread (page 168)
Watermelon
Lemonade or fruit juice
-or-
Pasta Shells with Crab &
    Mushrooms (page 123)
Banana Bran Muffins (page 170)
Cantaloupe filled with sliced
    strawberries
Ice tea
-or-
Rosemary-Scented Chicken Pilaf
    (page 104)
Banana-Apricot Bread (page 172)
Creamy Berry Ice (page 178)

To replace fluids after exercising, drink 2 cups of liquid for every pound lost through sweat. Any type of beverage or food with a high water content will help in rehydration. The exception to this rule is caffeinated beverages and alcohol. Both types of beverages act as a diuretic, causing the body to lose fluids instead of replacing them.

Q: My schedule is so hectic, I hardly have time to think about eating, much less have time to prepare nutritious meals. What are some general guidelines I can follow to make my diet healthier?

A: Eating regular balanced meals is a challenge for an active person with a busy schedule. Consider the following suggestions for making your calories count toward a healthier you:

• Eat something in the morning even if you have to take it with you. Some ideas include; granola cereal stirred into vanilla yogurt; a bagel spread with Neufchâtel cheese or a blender drink made with yogurt, fresh fruit and ice cubes.

• Drink plenty of fluids—8 to 10 glasses a day.

• Eat enough calories. Figure your caloric requirement by multiplying 17 times your present weight.

• Eat a balanced diet; never exclude any one food group. Eat at least half your calories in the form of carbohydrates such as grains, breads, cereals, pasta or starchy vegetables.

• Spread your calories evenly throughout the day. Your body works more efficiently with six small meals instead of one or two large ones.

• Pay special attention to your calcium and iron intake. A multivitamin with iron plus a calcium supplement may be advisable if you do not drink milk or eat much red meat.

WEIGHING THE ODDS

If exercising is not a regular part of your life, you may find yourself fighting an on-going battle of the bulge. Fatness is not fitness.

In our fast-paced automated society, Americans are eating less, yet are fatter than ever before. To combat this modern-day dilemma, many individuals enroll in some kind of weight-loss program, or try the latest diet on the newsstand. Diets are fine if the weight stays off—but it rarely does. Statistics show that 9 out of every 10 dieters regain their lost weight in less than 18 months.

Research is indicating that the "answer" to our nation's overweight problem is not to eat less, but to exercise more. This means building time into every day for physical activity—not just on the weekend, and committing to a consistent exercise routine. Intense, sporadic activity does not improve a person's conditioning, and rarely results in weight loss. On the other hand, perpetual dieting is not the answer either. It simply drains energy and produces spectators rather than participators.

MOVE IT & LOSE IT

The most important goal in weight loss is to reduce your body fat. A balanced diet and moderate exercise is the best way to do that. A person who loses weight by

ACTIVITY & CALORIE EXPENDITURE
(Figures based on a 150 pound individual per hour of activity)*

Walking (2 mph)	240
Bicycling (6 mph)	240
Rowing (2-1/2 mph)	300
Walking (3-1/2 mph)	330
Bicycling (8 mph)	330
Tennis	400
Aerobic dance	420
Recreational swimming	498
Running (5-1/2 mph)	600
Bicycling (13 mph)	600
Cross country skiing	700
Jogging (5-1/2 mph)	740
Jumping rope	950
Running (10 mph)	1020

*If you weigh 100 lbs., decrease calories by one-third. If you weigh 200 lbs., multiply calories by one and one-half.

Adapted from information from the American Heart Association.

dieting alone can actually lose more muscle than fat. Studies show that weight loss through dieting alone is about 75 percent fat and almost 25 percent lean muscle mass. Weight loss through a combination of diet and exercise, however, is about 98 percent fat and only 2 percent muscle weight. Since muscle burns more calories than fat, the more muscle you have, the more calories you burn even at rest.

Calorie expenditure is another advantage of exercise. You not only burn calories during the actual activity, but you burn more at rest after exercising than a non-active person. Research suggests that your basal metabolic rate (BMR) can increase as much as 10 percent for as long as 48 hours after exercise. So, instead of burning 80 calories an hour at rest, an active person would burn close to 90 calories per hour and would lose an extra 1/2 pound a week.

The number of calories burned during and after exercise depends on the intensity and duration of the activity. Generally speaking, the longer, less-intense types of exercise burn more fat calories than short bursts of activity. For example, jogging continuously for 40 minutes burns more calories than playing a game of doubles tennis for an hour. Approximately 100 calories are burned for every mile traveled by foot. For instance, your body burns about 300 calories whether you run 3 miles or walk 3 miles.

APPETITE SUPPRESSANT

Another benefit of exercise is that it may actually decrease appetite. Anyone who tries to eat after a hard workout knows that nothing is less appetizing than a large meal. Instead of increasing appetite, moderate exercise may actually make you feel less hungry.

EMOTIONAL WELL-BEING

Physically active people seem to benefit emotionally from exercise. A few minutes of aerobic-type activity each day makes the mind more calm and alert, reduces anxiety and may even be effective in treating depression.

Whether your exercise is a structured class at the spa or a brisk walk around the park, the important thing is to simply move more. Try to incorporate some type of playtime into your schedule every day.

FAT OR FIT

The definition of health, beauty and fitness has changed over the last 10 years. No longer is the gaunt emaciated look considered attractive. Today, the healthy, muscular, athletic look is more appealing. A heavy person is not necessarily fat, and a thin person is not necessarily fit. Beauty and fitness cannot be measured by a bathroom scale. Fitness is dependant on your percent of body fat.

An ideal percent of body fat for the average active male is 12 to 18 percent and 17 to 20 percent for a female.

ASSESSING BODY FAT

Of the several methods used in determining percentage of body fat, two common ways are the skinfold measurement and underwater (hydrostatic) weighing. Both methods are more reliable when done by someone who is experienced in taking skinfold measurements. Most health clubs and universities have trained personnel available who perform body assessments for the public. Check your local health club or sports medicine clinic for assistance. Skinfold measurements involve pinching the fat at different sites of your body with a small piece of equipment called skinfold calipers. The sum of the

BODY FAT	MEN	WOMEN
Essential	3%	13%
Average for the nonactive	15-18%	25-28%
Average for the active	10-15%	16-20%
Elite Athlete	5-8%	13-16%

Used with permission. Athlete's Kitchen, Nancy Clark, R.D., CBI Publishing Co., Boston, 1981.

various sites is then plugged into a series of mathematical equations to determine what percent of your total body weight is fat and what percent is muscle. From these calculations, an ideal weight is determined.

Underwater weighing is based on the Archimedean principle which, simply stated, says that fat floats. The technique involves weighing a person outside of water, then submerging him underwater and weighing again. By comparing dry weight to wet weight, your percent of body fat can be determined.

WHERE IS YOUR FAT?

Not only is the amount of fat you have important, but where your fat is deposited is also important. Increased fat accumulation around the waist, thigh and in the abdomen is associated with higher health risks, including diabetes and heart disease. Men, who accumulate fat around the waist, may be at higher risk than women who tend to accumulate fat in the thighs and hips.

The location of fat on the body also plays a role in its metabolic activity. Hip and thigh fat may be used to store fuel for energy, and seems to become more metabolically active at different times during a person's life. For instance, a woman who is pregnant or lactating tends to use the fat stored on her hips and thighs for energy.

Be patient with yourself when trying to lose fat weight. It probably takes a good six weeks of regular exercise and eating less calories to notice a change in body fat.

WEIGHT GAIN THEORIES

If you have ever tried to lose weight, you know how frustrating it is to try and attain an ideal percent of body fat. Sometimes cutting back on calories and exercising more just is not enough. Why can some people eat whatever they want and never gain weight, while others gain weight by breathing deeply while standing in a bakery? The cause or causes of obesity are not clearly understood, but research suggests several theories which may play a role in the weight problem.

Set Point Theory

One theory proposes that the human body will, if not manipulated, seek out its own natural weight or "set point."

This set point may be higher for obese individuals than for the normal population. According to this theory it is very difficult for an obese person to lose and maintain an ideal weight when his natural weight is set at 10 to 20 pounds heavier than is recommended.

Slow Metabolism Theory

A sluggish metabolism may be another contributing factor to the obesity picture. Some individuals tend to need fewer calories for normal body functions than the average person. This slower basal metabolic rate (BMR) is influenced by several factors, such as age, gender, size, hormones and nutritional status. A young person has a higher metabolism than an older person. A man generally requires more calories than a woman because of both his larger size and greater percent of muscle mass. Abnormal hormonal levels from the thyroid, adrenal and pituitary glands can also result in a slower metabolism.

Brown Fat Theory

A small percentage of body weight is composed of brown fat that is located in specific areas of the body. This fat may be an important factor in burning excess calories. The Brown Fat Theory proposes that a lean person may have extra or more effective brown fat than an obese person. Theoretically, the more brown fat a person has, the more calories he burns, and the less he weighs. Unfortunately, brown fat seems to be genetically determined. If it's not in your genes, you cannot produce brown fat, no matter how hard you try. For an individual who is genetically predisposed to brown fat, it can be triggered into use by two things—exposure to the cold and ingestion of food. It seems to become less functional with age.

Fat Cell Theory

Lastly, the Fat Cell Theory suggests that when a person loses weight, his fat cells become smaller, but they still exist. These depleted fat cells may send signals to the brain and cause a person to actually feel hungrier at a lower weight. According to this theory, a person can still reduce his weight by modifying his diet, but he may have trouble keeping the weight off because the smaller fat cells are telling his brain that he is hungry. The more weight he loses, the hungrier he feels.

WAYS TO BATTLE YOUR BULGE: STARVATION

Many times dieting means starvation, but it does not work. If you severely restrict your calories, you will actually gain weight. Undereating promotes obesity by fooling the body into conserving energy. When food is restricted, your body turns down its thermostat, so to speak, and operates on as few calories as possible.

WATER WEIGHT

Another problem associated with severe restriction of food is a situation referred to as "refeeding edema." If you start eating normally again after a strict diet, you will retain more water than usual. The "yo-yo" effect common to many dieters is often related to water retention and water loss, as opposed to an increase and decrease in fat weight.

BINGING

The more you diet, usually the more you eat when you get the chance. Studies suggest that a person who consciously restricts his calories tends to eat more when he finally does allow himself to eat. His appetite seems insatiable: the more he eats, the hungrier he becomes.

NO-DIET DIET

Obviously, starvation doesn't work. Neither do any of the other so called "popcorn" diets that are so popular among those who want a quick fix, an easy answer to their weight problem. A "popcorn" diet is based on a kernal of truth, but it is blown full of hot air by someone selling some kind of pill or secret formula. The most effective weight loss program incorporates diet, exercise, and behavior modification. An effective weight control and fitness program will include the following principles:

- Eat small portions
- Eat more often
- Get a good start
- Exercise more often

Eat Small Portions

When you are trying to lose weight, never totally eliminate any one food group; simply cut down on the amount that you eat. For example, when eating at a Mexican food restaurant, order a la carte instead of getting a full meal. Instead of a whole piece of pie, cut it in half and share it with a friend. To further decrease calories, try substituting a food that is lower in calories. For instance, low-fat plain yogurt tastes very similar to sour cream, yet has fewer calories and less fat.

Eat More Often

Another key to losing fat is to eat more often. Many of us with hectic lifestyles tend to eat one meal a day, convinced that we are saving on total calories and losing weight. Research shows, however, that more fat accumulates when you eat one large meal instead of spreading those same calories throughout the day. Try to eat four to six times a day—three small meals with one or two small snacks.

Getting a Good Start

How important is eating breakfast? Eating something in the morning will make you more alert, increase your energy level and keep you from snacking late at night. Despite popular thinking, a person saves very few calories when he skips breakfast. Studies suggest that breakfast-skippers tend to consume the calories later in the day, usually before bed. You probably know someone who eats a 500 calorie snack before bed, but absolutely refuses a 300-calorie breakfast on the grounds he is trying to lose weight.

Eating breakfast can actually reduce body fat. One of my patients, Tom, was losing 2 to 3 pounds consistently each week on a combined exercise and diet program. The problem was that the weight he was losing was coming from muscle instead of fat. A review of his food records showed that he skipped breakfast at least 5 times a week. Tom agreed to include breakfast every day for a month. He continued to lose 2 to 3 pounds a week, but most of the weight lost was coming from fat stores instead of lean muscle mass.

Many people claim they feel hungrier at mid-morning if they eat breakfast, than if they skip it. One reason for this is the increase in metabolism associated with eating a meal. Breakfast may start your gastric juices flowing, making you feel hungry. In the long run, however, it probably prevents you from overeating at lunch or later in the day.

Breakfast does not have to be the

LO-CAL FOOD SUBSTITUTES

FOOD ITEM	SUBSTITUTE	CALORIC SAVINGS
Syrup-packed canned peaches	Water-packed canned peaches	62 cal/cup
Cream cheese	Neufchâtel cheese	30 cal/oz.
Whole milk	Skim milk	68 cal/cup
Ice cream	Ice milk	58 cal/cup
Whipped cream	Evaporated skim milk, whipped	106 cal/1/2 cup
Canned bouillon	Bouillon granules	25 cal/cup
Sour cream	Yogurt, low-fat	270 cal/cup
Cheddar cheese	Mozzarella or Farmer's cheese	20 cal/oz.
Sausage	Ground beef	491 cal/pound
Sandwich bread	Extra-thin bread	35 cal/slice
Butter crackers	Saltine crackers	5 cal/cracker
Fruit flavored yogurt	Plain low-fat yogurt plus 1 tablespoon sugar and 1/3 cup fruit	30 cal/cup
10 Tortilla chips	1 cup unbuttered, popped popcorn	120 cal

traditional bacon and eggs. Choose any type of food that is high in fiber, and provides some fat and protein that will "stick" with you throughout the morning. Some breakfast ideas include:

• Spread a rice cake with 1 teaspoon peanut butter.

• Blend 1 egg, 6 ounces low-fat plain yogurt, 2 tablespoons frozen orange juice concentrate and ice cubes until smooth.

• Put a layer of whole grain cereal, such as granola, in the bottom of a parfait dish. Top with vanilla yogurt and fresh fruit such as blueberries, strawberries or bananas. Repeat the layers.

• Spread 1/2 of an English muffin with 2 teaspoons of low-fat ricotta cheese. Sprinkle with cinnamon and broil 2 to 3 minutes, or until warm. Top with sliced canned or fresh fruit such as strawberries, bananas, mandarin oranges or peaches.

• Fill a baked apple with raisins and top with a granola-type cereal. Warm in the microwave.

• Cereal—both hot and cold—is a popular option for a quick nutritious breakfast. Most cereals are loaded with vitamins, minerals and fiber. Look for the enriched varieties of cold cereal that have very little added sugar such as Cheerios,

Chex cereals, Shredded Wheat, Total, Special K and Product 19, to name a few.

To add variety to a cooked cereal, try the following suggestions.

• Cook hot cereal in low-fat or skim milk instead of water.

• When cooking hot cereal, add 2 tablespoons of non-fat dry milk powder or an egg white and increase the protein content substantially.

• Top hot cereal with fresh bananas, canned peaches, applesauce or granola.

• For a sweeter flavor, add raisins, dates or dried apples to cooked cereal.

Munch a Lunch

If you pack a lunch, start early. Make your sandwich ahead of time and freeze it. Take the sandwich from the freezer in the morning before school or work, and it should be thawed by lunch. To add some variety to the standard sandwich, try different kinds of bread such as pumpernickel, pocket bread, bagel, onion roll or Date Bran Bread, page 173.

Bored with sandwiches? You can pack the filling separately to eat with crackers, tortillas or lavosh. Some different sandwich fillings include:

• Neufchâtel cheese mixed with green onion and cucumber. Or, mix dates and raisins with the cheese and spread on a bagel.

- Pocket bread filled with tuna salad. Mix the tuna with grated carrot, celery and chopped pimiento and moisten with a mixture of low-fat yogurt and reduced calorie mayonnaise.
- Try the Skagway Salmon, page 58 for a different luncheon treat.
- Another tasty sandwich can be made with Mushroom-Veal Loaf, page 88.

If you plan to freeze a sandwich filling, remember that some fillings freeze better than others. Fillings that do not freeze well include foods such as eggs, mayonnaise, jelly, lettuce or tomatoes.

If your time for lunch is limited, consider the following suggestions for a quick meal.

- Stuffed vegetables. Stuff a tomato or red bell pepper with cottage cheese or tuna salad. A green bell pepper stuffed with Tabbuli, page 155 is an especially good take-along lunch.
- Soup—cold or hot—packed in a thermos. Try the Blender Gazpacho Soup, page 69.

- Breast of chicken. Poach several chicken breasts at one time and refrigerate to use for a quick lunch later in the week. Chop the meat and toss it with cooked vegetables and a light dressing for a main-dish salad.
- Meat and vegetables that are left over from a previous meal make a great stir-fry dish if you eat lunch at home.
- Sprinkle shredded part-skim Swiss cheese in a pocket-bread half, wrap in a paper towel and microwave until cheese melts. Open the sandwich and stuff with a mixture of alfalfa sprouts, red bell pepper, celery and a light vinaigrette salad dressing.
- Spread an English muffin half with pureed cottage cheese and top with prepared pizza sauce. Arrange fresh vegetable slices such as red bell pepper, green bell pepper and mushrooms on top of the pizza sauce. Sprinkle with grated mozzarella cheese; bake at 450F (230C) about 5 minutes.

A sample menu is provided below for you to get an idea of what a nutritious low-calorie meal plan would look like.

		CALORIES
BREAKFAST:	1 slice raisin toast with	66
	1 teaspoon margarine	45
	6 ounces vanilla yogurt	146
	1 fresh orange	60
	1/3 cup granola cereal (mixed with yogurt)	126
LUNCH:	Turkey sandwich:	
	3 ounces turkey	180
	2 whole-wheat bread slices	140
	1 teaspoon mayonnaise	45
	Lettuce, tomato	5
	Carrot and celery sticks	20
	1 cup 2% milk	120
DINNER:	Spaghetti and meatballs (10 ounces homemade)	396
	Tossed salad with a variety of vegetables	70
	1 tablespoon salad dressing	80
	1 French bread slice	80
	1 teaspoon margarine	45
	Iced tea	0
	1 cup fresh sliced strawberries	162
	Total	1846

Snacks

If you have a habit of reaching for a processed snack food like potato chips, try stocking your kitchen with the following foods:

- Raw vegetables cleaned and stored in a plastic bag in the refrigerator.
- Popcorn prepared with a minimal amount of butter-flavored salt.
- Fresh fruit, washed and stored in a plastic bag in the refrigerator.
- Rice cakes or rice crackers.
- On the weekend, prepare your favorite dip and store it in the refrigerator for a quick snack with fresh vegetables later in the week.

GETTING STARTED—HOW TO MAXIMIZE YOUR TIME

Begin a lifetime of well-being by taking charge of your health. Take control of your eating habits. Take time to plan your meals, learn about food labels, organize your kitchen and learn some cooking techniques that save time and energy.

Even with best intentions, healthy cooking is a challenge for anyone who feels the pinch of time. If you buy foods that are preprepared, you should know which are the best buy for your dollar. If you eat on the run, you should know which fast foods are the most nutritious and how to order in a restaurant so you fill up and not out.

ORGANIZE YOUR KITCHEN

Menu planning is important if you are serious about taking control of your health. To help you get started, consider the following suggestions:

- Plan meals for several days or a week in advance so you can compile one grocery list and avoid last minute confusion over what to serve.
- Shop for groceries once a week. Instead of daily runs to the supermarket, use the time to run around the tennis court a few extra times during the week.
- Simplify your meals. Limit your meals to 2 or 3 uncomplicated courses. An example of a streamlined dinner is a meat and vegetable stir-fry served with rice. Conclude your meal with Fruit & Berry Gratin on page 175.
- Count on leftovers when planning meals. Cooked meat, poultry or fish can be ground for a sandwich filling or chopped and added to soups, casseroles or salads.
- Plan dishes that require a minimal amount of preparation. For instance, serve a cantaloupe half filled with green grapes instead of a sliced fruit cup for dessert.
- Be prepared. For last minute meals, stock your kitchen with basics foods such as:

Breads: pasta, rice, dry stuffing mix, flour or corn tortillas, frozen bread dough.

Fruits: assortment of canned, fresh or frozen fruit—peaches, applesauce, apples, oranges, bananas.

Vegetables: assortment of canned, fresh, or frozen vegetables, tomatoes and tomato products, garlic, onions.

Dairy: plain low-fat yogurt, canned evaporated skim milk, low-fat cheese.

Protein: water-packed tuna, eggs, peanut butter.

Miscellaneous: Picante sauce, olive oil, vinegar, vegetable spray, assorted spices and herbs.

READING LABELS

To cook healthy, you have to buy healthy. Knowing how to read food labels will help. Labeling is a useful tool for evaluating details about a product such as the cost, nutrient value and specific ingredients it contains.

If trying to read labels has you frustrated, don't despair. The terminology that manufacturers use to sell their products is unclear at best. For instance according to the Food and Drug Administration (FDA), which supervises most grocery foods, the word *natural* on a label has no meaning. In other words, food manufacturers can devise their own definition for it because legally there is no guideline for what natural means.

There are some regulations, however, regarding food labels. A few terms like low-calorie or low-sodium are specifically defined by the FDA. If a manufacturer makes a specific health claim about a product, the package must contain complete nutrition information to support that claim. Ingredients must be listed in descending order according to the percentage of weight the ingredient contributes to the total product. And, lastly, misleading photographs on food products are against the law.

To help you evaluate packaged foods and make sense of labels, refer to the glossary below:

• Diet or dietetic: Read the label carefully. Unless stated otherwise, these products must contain no more than 40 calories per serving or have at least 1/3 fewer calories than the regular product.

• Enriched or fortified: In terms of labeling, these words have the same meaning, the product contains added protein, vitamins or minerals. The label must specifically list the nutrients added and give the amount of each nutrient per serving.

• Imitation: This word indicates that the product is nutritionally inferior to the real product. For example, "imitation cheese" has less calories and protein than real cheese. Foods that are not the real thing, but are nutritionally equal to the food they are imitating are labeled *substitute*.

• Light or lite: A questionable word. These products usually contain fewer calories and fat, but may be light only in texture or color. If a label says "light" and elaborates with specific terms like "one half the fat," the claims must be substantiated in the fine print on the label. Without specific claims, a product labeled light is probably only different in appearance.

• Low-calorie: These foods must contain no more than 40 calories per serving or 0.4 calories per gram.

• Low-fat: Legally, this term applies only to meat and dairy products. The FDA requires that low-fat dairy products must contain between 0.5 percent and 2 percent milk fat. Low-fat meat, however, must have no more than 10 percent fat by weight.

• Natural: As mentioned earlier, the FDA does not define the term "natural." The United States Department of Agriculture (USDA)—which monitors meat—does define natural to mean that there are no artificial colors, flavors, preservatives or synthetic ingredients of any kind in the meat or poultry.

• No cholesterol: Don't be mislead by this claim. A low-cholesterol product may still contain saturated fat and can be just as unhealthy as cholesterol.

• Organic: This is another term without legal definition. A manufacturer can create his own meaning and use the term without any guidelines.

• Sodium-free: A product that has less than 5 mg of sodium per serving is considered sodium-free. A "very low-sodium" product must have no more than 35 mg per serving. "Low-salt" products must contain no more than 140 mg of sodium per serving. Beware of the term "no salt added." Although no salt is added to a product during processing, the food may be naturally high in sodium and is therefore not necessarily salt-free.

• Sugar-free or sugarless: Be careful of this term. Foods may not contain any table sugar, but may have other sweeteners such as honey, corn syrup, fructose, sorbitol or mannitol added. Read the label carefully to see if the product is truly lower in calories.

What Is on a Nutrition Label?

Nutrition information on a label is divided into two categories: Nutritional Information Per Serving and Percentage of the United States Recommended Daily Allowance (US RDA).

Nutrition Information Per Serving includes serving size, servings per container, protein, carbohydrate and fat in grams per serving. The amount of sodium per serving is also included. The label described opposite is from a box of yellow corn meal.

The information in the second category—Percentage of US RDA—must include the amounts of protein, vitamin A, vitamin C, thiamin, niacin, riboflavin, calcium and iron. A sample label is shown below.

A list of ingredients is required by law for most packaged foods. Those that do not require a complete ingredient list include fresh meat, fruits, vegetables, poultry and fish. Some products may only list the optional ingredients such as flavorings or emulsifiers. Products that have the same ingredients regardless of the manufacturer are regulated by a term called "Standard of Identity." Such products as ice cream, ketchup and mayonnaise do not have their ingredients listed on the label.

Read labels carefully and question

YELLOW CORN MEAL

SERVING SIZE
    Serving Size, About 3 tablespoons, 1 oz. (28 g)

SERVING SIZE tells the specific quantity on which the nutrition information is based.

SERVINGS PER CONTAINER   24

SERVINGS PER CONTAINER tells how many people you can expect to serve. It also helps in calculating cost per serving: Divide the cost of the container by the number of servings. For example:
$4.00 ÷ 8 servings per container = $.50 per serving

NUTRITION INFORMATION PER SERVING

CALORIES	100
PROTEIN	2 g
CARBOHYDRATE	22 g
FAT	1 g

SODIUM WHEN PREPARED WITHOUT SALT
    Not more than 10 mg per serving

POTASSIUM	45 mg

SODIUM. Sodium labeling is required by law, and is expressed in mg per serving.

OPTIONAL INFORMATION supplied voluntarily by the manufacturer on other vitamins and minerals, cholesterol, types of fats and carbohydrates.

INGREDIENTS: Degerminated yellow corn meal, niacin, reduced iron, thiamin mononitrate, riboflavin.

INGREDIENTS are listed in order of percentage that they are present in the product. Food additives are listed, but specific names do not have to be named.

PERCENTAGE OF THE U.S. RECOMMENDED DAILY ALLOWANCES (US RDA)

PER 1 OZ. SERVING

Protein	2
Vitamin A	*
Vitamin C	*
Thiamin	8
Riboflavin	4
Niacin	4
Calcium	*
Iron	4

NUTRITION INFORMATION is expressed as a percent of the US RDA for protein, five vitamins and two minerals. Additional information may also be found here, such as additional vitamins, cholesterol, types of fat and types of carbohydrate.

*Contains less than 2% of the US RDA for this nutrient. For additional nutritional information, write to Consumer Response, The Quaker Oats Company, Chicago, IL 60654

Name and place of business of either the manufacturer or distributor must be on the label. This is the address to send questions or comments about the product. Telephone numbers are also included on some labels.

the manufacturer's claims and marketing tactics. Beware of colors on labels, catchy phrases and old-fashioned lettering on packages; they may or may not have any similarity to the actual product. Ask yourself if the claims make sense. Phrases like "no preservatives" are unnecessary for foods such as jams, jellies or orange juice. "No artificial flavors" doesn't necessarily mean no artificial color or preservatives. Evaluate a product thoroughly before making food choices based upon labeling claims.

ORGANIZING YOUR KITCHEN

Stocking your kitchen with a variety of foods and time-saving equipment makes cooking nutritious meals a snap.

Equipment

• A food processor or electric blender. A food processor chops the vegetables for Mushroom Caviar, page 54, in only seconds. A blender is great for pureeing vegetables for "cream" soup without the cream or for whirling up the Quick Banana Shake, on page 197.

• A wok, a nonstick pan, a broiling pan with drain holes, parchment paper and poultry shears will help you avoid unwanted fat in your cooking.

• A steamer or microwave-safe cookware will help retain important nutrients in your food.

• A complete set of freezer-proof containers.

Aside from equipment, you should know how to make convenience foods from your own kitchen. The following list will help get you started.

Fruits & Vegetables

• Cut up vegetables as soon as you get home from the market. Celery, carrots and bell pepper that are cut into match-sized pieces take no time to throw into a salad or stir-fry dish.

• When cooking with onion, chop the entire onion and freeze the unused portion in a freezer-proof container. Frozen chopped onions are great for soups and sauces or for sauteeing with other vegetables.

• Spoon unused portions of tomato paste in tablespoon-size amounts onto a cookie sheet and freeze. When frozen, place the tomato paste in a plastic bag and store it in the freezer for use in sauces and for flavoring stews or soups.

• When squeezing fresh lemons or oranges for juice, first grate the peel, taking care to remove only the outer colored portion of the peel. Wrap teaspoon portions in freezer paper and freeze.

Dairy

• Grate cheese used for cooking soon after you get home from the supermarket. Grated cheese keeps in the freezer for several months and is especially good to use in baked dishes.

Meats

• After poaching a chicken, pour any cooled, unused stock into an ice-cube tray and freeze. When firm, put the frozen cubes in a plastic bag and store them in the freezer. This is a great low-sodium alternative for canned chicken broth or chicken bouillon.

• For quick barbecued chicken, bake a whole cut-up chicken with the skin on and refrigerate the pieces. To barbecue: remove the skin, brush with barbecue sauce and place the chicken on the grill. Cook it until warmed thoroughly—about 20 minutes.

• Slice flank steak for stir-fry, or cube a beef roast for kebabs immediately after you get home from the market. Put the meat in a freezer-proof bag and store in the freezer until the day before you plan to use it. Remove the bag from the freezer and place it in a mixing bowl. Pour your favorite marinade directly over the meat in the bag and set it in the refrigerator to thaw and marinate at the same time.

• For quick grilled fish, rub fish fillets with olive, almond or sesame oil, pat with fresh herbs such as basil, oregano or tarragon. Grill over mesquite wood.

• Use your microwave for a head start on a dish that requires many steps to prepare. Partially cook meats, poultry, potatoes or casseroles first in the microwave, then finish the cooking in a conventional oven.

Grains & Cereals

• Freeze bread and tortillas that you are not using right away.

- When you prepare beans, legumes or rice, cook 3 to 4 times the quantity you need and freeze the unused amount in serving-size portions. Reheat in the microwave and use the rice or legumes as a side dish, or mix it with chopped vegetables and meat for a complete meal.
- Freeze Marinara Sauce, page 138, in 1/4- to 1/2-cup quantities. To prepare: Thaw in the microwave, or put the sauce in a casserole dish and thaw in a warm oven. Boil some pasta and toss with the thawed sauce. You can have a delicious side dish in the time it takes to boil some noodles.
- Slice French bread into serving-size portions. Wrap in freezer-proof foil and freeze it until just before you are ready to serve. Put it in a warm oven to thaw 15 minutes before dinner.

Planning ahead is not only important for meals you cook at home, but it is also beneficial when you eat away from home.

EATING ON THE RUN

At least 46 million Americans eat in a fast food restaurant every day. Our hectic lifestyles make eating in a hurry par for the course. Fast food restaurants provide fast foods for fast times, but do they provide nutritious food for active bodies?

Generally speaking, fast foods supply adequate amounts of protein and B vitamins, but they are high in salt and fat. Many times fast foods are low in calcium and vitamins A and C. To increase the nutrient value of fast food, try the suggestions below:

- When ordering a hamburger, leave off the cheese. It adds 406 mg sodium, 106 extra calories and 9 grams fat.
- Include low-fat milk as a beverage instead of soft drinks, coffee or tea. Although diet soft drinks, black coffee and unsweetened tea are calorie-free, they do not contribute the calcium that milk does.
- Be adventuresome. Try the new salads available at many fast-food restaurants. Look for salads that contain vitamin-packed vegetables such as tomato, green bell pepper, spinach and carrots.
- Include juice at breakfast when possible. Three-fourths cup of orange, grapefruit or tomato juice supplies at least 100 percent of the US RDA for vitamin C.

Is Faster Always Fatter?

Because you have no way to control the ingredients, restaurant food is probably higher in fat than homemade. An average cheeseburger at a fast food restaurant contains the equivalent of 11 teaspoons of margarine. Fried foods, mayonnaise or mayonnaise-based condiments, high fat meats and pastries all contribute a substantial amount of fat to a restaurant meal. To avoid the quantity of fat when you eat out, try the following suggestions:

- When ordering a salad, limit the amount of salad dressing you use.
- When ordering sandwich-type items, leave off the mayonnaise or mayonnaise-based condiment. Try spicy mustard or reduced-calorie Italian salad dressing instead.
- Avoid cream soups—order broth-based soups instead.
- Order sour cream, margarine, salad dressing, tartar sauce, mayonnaise and grated cheese on the side, and add it to your food yourself.
- Limit the amount of flaky pastries you eat. An occasional treat is fine, but they are too high in fat to eat on a regular basis. The very flakiness that makes a pastry taste so good is directly related to the amount of fat it contains.
- Choose meats that are lower in fat. A London broil is leaner than prime rib. Order baked, roasted or broiled chicken and fish.
- Limit fried foods, such as fried potatoes, fried chicken or fish sandwiches and fried desserts.They may be fried in a highly saturated fat.
- Avoid added cheese. A baked potato with cheese sauce from a fast-food restaurant contains the equivalent of 3 tablespoons margarine.
- If you eat breakfast away from home, avoid high-fat meats like bacon or sausage. Leaner breakfast items include foods such as plain biscuits, pancakes, English muffins and bagels.

Refer to the chart on page 45 for specific guidelines in making lean fast food choices.

A Fat Is a Fat Is a Fat—Or Is It?

Not only is the quantity of fat we eat a concern, but the type of fat we eat is also important. In recent years, you have probably heard a lot about fast-food restaurants using beef tallow to fry their foods. What are the major health concerns associated with beef tallow?

The main problem with beef tallow is that it is extremely saturated and contains cholesterol. The more saturated the fat, generally speaking, the greater the effect it has in raising blood cholesterol. Some restaurant chains use different oils at different outlets. Ask your particular fast-food outlet what type of fat they use for frying. If vegetable oil is used, ask if it is either moderately or heavily hydrogenated. Hydrogenation is a chemical process which makes a vegetable oil saturated. If you eat fried foods, those fried in moderately hydrogenated oil are better than foods fried in heavily hydrogenated oil or beef tallow. To find out more about the specific nutrient content of your favorite fast-foods, ask at the particular outlet, or see page 201 for a list of addresses you can write for more information.

TAKE-OUT FOOD FROM YOUR SUPERMARKET

To meet the consumer demand for added convenience, many supermarkets offer expanded delicatessen items and a selection of warm foods that are available for take-out. In addition to the traditional meats and cheeses, many delis have cold seafood salads, pasta salads and vegetable salads. The shaved ham, turkey and roast beef in the delicatessen of your supermarket are good to have on hand for a quick sandwich. These meats are usually leaner than packaged lunch meats.

The warm take-out food are freshly prepared entrees that are ready to eat as purchased. The advantage to this type of food is that the ingredients are fresh, the processing is minimal and the food is ready to eat without further preparation. You can stop at the supermarket on your way home from work and have the majority of your meal ready when you arrive home. Add a tossed salad or fresh fruit and a beverage to make a complete meal.

Roast chicken is available at many supermarkets, and is a very versatile choice if you don't have time to cook a chicken at home. You can skin and slice it for a traditional roast chicken dinner. Or,

you can skin it and chop the meat for any recipe that calls for cooked chicken.

Buying at least one part of your meal precooked saves time and energy, without necessarily compromising its nutritional quality. The advantage of take-out food from a supermarket as compared to take-out food from a restaurant, is that there is a greater selection of foods, you don't have to call ahead to place an order and it is usually less expensive.

FROZEN DINNERS: HOW DO THEY RATE?

Commercially prepared frozen dinners are fast becoming standard fare for young working Americans. During the last five years, the typical TV dinner has taken on a new identity. Frozen fried chicken, mashed potatoes and green peas have evolved into every ethnic dish imaginable that is either fat-controlled, calorie-controlled or ready-to-eat in less than 10 minutes. Let's take a look at these frozen meals and see how they compare in fat, calories, salt, nutrients and cost.

Calorie Controlled

Some of the early versions of reduced-calorie frozen dinners contained 400 to 700 calories per serving. The newer versions are closer to 250 to 300 calories per serving.

These low-calorie dinners are great for a person who expends an average amount of energy each day. For a very active person, however, these dinners are more like a snack. For example, if you eat 1800 calories a day, a reduced calorie dinner would provide only 14 percent of the energy that you need each day. To boost the calories and nutrient content of these meals, add some low-fat cottage cheese, a large dinner roll and a tossed salad made with plenty of tomatoes and carrots.

Fat-Controlled

Many of the reduced-calorie dinners are also lower in fat, but not all of them. Read the labels carefully. Look for the total number of grams of fat per serving, as opposed to the percentage of fat calories. Frequently, with low-calorie foods, the percentage of fat looks higher than what is recommended because there are so few calories. For example, a frozen dinner may have only 11 grams of fat per

	CALORIES	TOTAL FAT (gm)	FAT (% of calories)
McDONALD'S			
Hamburger	225	10	35
Chicken McNuggets	314	19	54
Filet-O-Fish	432	25	52
Big Mac	563	33	53
Sausage Biscuit	582	40	61
WENDY'S			
Pasta Salad (1/2 cup)	134	6	40
Chicken Sandwich on Wheat Bun	320	10	28
Taco Salad	390	18	40
Broccoli and Cheese Potato	500	25	45
Cheese Stuffed Potato	590	34	52
HARDEE'S			
Chef's Salad	272	16	53
Chicken Fillet Sandwich	510	26	46
Shrimp Salad	362	29	72
Bacon Cheeseburger	686	42	55
ARBY'S			
Roast Chicken Breast (no bun)	254	7	25
Broccoli Cheese Potato	540	22	37
Mushroom and Cheese Potato	510	22	39
Fried Chicken Breast Sandwich	584	28	43
Sausage and Egg Croissant	530	35	59
LONG JOHN SILVER'S			
Baked Fish with sauce	151	2	12
Mixed Vegetables	54	2	33
Corn-on-the-cob	176	4	20
Coleslaw	182	15	74
Fish with batter (2 pc.)	404	24	53
BURGER KING			
Veal Parmigiana	580	27	42
Bacon Double Cheeseburger	600	35	53
Specialty Chicken Sandwich	690	42	55
JACK IN THE BOX			
Shrimp Salad (no dressing)	115	1	8
Taco Salad	377	24	57
Chicken Supreme Salad	601	36	54
KENTUCKY FRIED CHICKEN			
Breast (original recipe)	199	12	53
Extra Crispy Dark Dinner	765	54	63

Reprinted from *Nutrition Action Healthletter*, which is available from the Center for Science in the Public Interest, 1501 16th Street, NW, Washington, D.C. 20036, for $19.95 for 10 issues. Copyright 1988.

serving, but those 11 grams comprise 41 percent of the total 250 calories. Buy frozen dinners with 10 to 15 grams of fat per serving.

The following guidelines may help you in choosing a low-fat frozen food:

LEAN: A dinner is considered lean if it has 15 or less grams of fat per serving. Some products that fall into this category include Great Escapes Lite Entrees, Armour Dinner Classics, La Choy, Light and Elegant, Stouffer's Lean Cuisine, Benihana and Mrs. Paul's Light Seafood Entrees.

MODERATELY LEAN: Moderately lean dinners have 15 to 20 grams of fat per serving and include brands such as Weight Watchers Frozen Entrees, Chung King, Green Giant, Le Menu and Stouffer's Entrees.

HIGH-FAT: Entrees that have 20 or more grams of fat per serving are considered high-fat. These products include Swanson Four-Part Dinners, Patio Dinners, Hungry Man Dinners, Old El Paso and some Budget Gourmet Dinners.

Salt

Most frozen entrees average about 1000 mg of sodium per serving. The significance of the sodium contained in a dish depends on how much salt is eaten during the rest of the day. The recommendation for salt intake is 1100 to 3300 mg per day. One meal that contains 1000 to 2000 mg of sodium is not necessarily excessive if the other foods eaten during the day are low in salt. Read the label on your favorite frozen dinner to determine the salt content. Stouffer's Beef Chop Suey is one dinner that tops the chart at 2000 mg per serving. On the other hand, Old El Paso frozen dishes average about 625 mg of sodium per serving.

Nutrients

Frozen dinners vary widely in their nutrient content. Unless a product is actually labeled "dinner", it is probably low in vitamins A and C. Products that contain a substantial amount of these vitamins include brands such as Banquet American Favorite Dinners, Armour Dinner Classics, Classic Lites and Le Menu.

Most frozen entrees provide only 10 percent of the US RDA for calcium. If you choose these products, include a low-fat dairy food at the same meal. Some ideas might include grilled cheese bread made with low-fat cheese, a salad tossed with grated Parmesan cheese, or a fruit salad with yogurt dressing. A glass of skim or 2 percent milk is a great way to add some calcium to your diet.

Many frozen entrees are low in thiamin, riboflavin and iron. The way to boost these nutrients is to add some kind of enriched grain product such as rice, noodles, bulgur salad or a pasta side-dish. Try Gazpacho Rice Salad, page 156, for a delicious complement to a frozen dish that is low in B vitamins and iron.

To evaluate frozen convenience foods, read the label carefully. Keep your eye out for new, innovative products. A few companies are trying new ways to increase the nutrients and reduce the sodium and fat. They are using tofu, low-fat cheese and more vegetables in their products. Some companies are trying to use fewer additives, which are probably not harmful to health, but which lessen the quality and taste of the food. The variety and selection of these products will only improve with time.

Paying the Price

Many individuals, especially young professionals, are willing to pay any price to stay out of the kitchen. Buying frozen dinners is one way to accomplish this objective. The cost of these frozen meals is about four times the cost of the fresh ingredients. Packaging and advertising increases the cost. Some lower-priced products include brands such as Stouffer's Entrees, Budget Gourmet, Banquet and Swanson Dinners.

HOMEMADE FROZEN ENTREES

Making your own frozen dinners is one way to ensure quick nutritious meals. With a little planning, you can have convenience foods from your own freezer at about one-fourth the cost of commercially prepared frozen dinners. For the best success in freezing foods, keep in mind the following suggestions:

● Remove all the air from the freezer bag before sealing.

● Use only freezer-proof wrap and moisture-proof containers. Cool food thoroughly before freezing.

• Remember that liquids expand when frozen, so allow about 1/2-inch space at the top of the container when freezing soups, stews and sauces.

• Foods that do not freeze well include fried foods, lettuce, tomatoes, celery, cucumber, radishes and potatoes. Casserole dishes that contain small amounts of the above ingredients will freeze fine.

• Do not put aluminum foil directly over acidic foods like tomato sauce. The acid can eat a hole in the aluminum. The food will no longer be tightly sealed, and will freezer burn.

• To freeze berries such as blueberries, strawberries, raspberries and blackberries, place the whole fruit in a single layer on the bottom of a shallow-rimmed pan and freeze. When firm, remove the fruit from the pan and place in a freezer bag. Return to the freezer. Fruit frozen in this way is great for making blender drinks.

• If you plan to cook your frozen meals in the microwave, freeze them in a plastic, glass or microwave-safe container. Arrange the food in shallow layers for quicker reheating.

• Cover a dish to be microwaved with plastic wrap, and loosen the covering or put holes in it before heating.

• Plan on 5 or 7 minutes of microwave cooking time at the High setting for individual-sized dinners.

PUTTING IT ALL TOGETHER

Eating to stay fit is a challenge for anyone. Fortunately, you can do it if you make it a priority. Some steps to help you get started in cooking, looking and feeling your best are included below:

• Tune into your health objective. Determine the area of your diet that you would like to work on the most, and develop a plan of action from there. For instance, if fat is getting the upper hand in your diet, write down on a piece of paper that your health goal is to decrease the amount of fat that you are presently eating.

• With your health objective in mind, take stock of your present eating habits and be realistic in your expectations of how you want to achieve your goal. Your eating habits have taken a lifetime to establish; you cannot expect to "undo" the negative ones overnight.

• Incorporate sound nutritional knowledge into what you are already doing. For instance, if you enjoy and eat meat frequently, simply modify the type and amount of meat that you eat. Don't exclude it entirely from your meal plans.

• Expect to change or modify your eating habits gradually. For example, if ice cream is a daily indulgence for you, try frozen yogurt or sorbet instead, and reduce your fat intake substantially. Strawberry Sorbet on page 179 is a great frozen dessert with the creaminess and all the flavor of regular ice cream, but with none of the fat. Adapt your favorite recipes and food preferences to the techniques and ingredients you know are nutritionally sound. Ask yourself how your recipes can be prepared along the lines of less sugar, fat and salt and with more fiber. For example: "Is it necessary to saute the onions in butter? Do the muffins need all that sugar?" An example of how to turn a traditional recipe into a lean version is shown on page 48.

Keep in mind the following cooking tips when modifying your recipes:

• The fresher the ingredients, the better. Simplify the cooking techniques to minimize fat and calories.

• Instead of sour cream, blend low-fat cottage cheese with plain low-fat yogurt until smooth.

• Substitute tomato juice for all or part of the oil when preparing commercial French-style salad dressing mixes.

• Use evaporated skim milk to dip foods in before breading for baking.

• Use bouillon cubes for seasoning cooked vegetables instead of butter.

• Use part-skim milk cheeses

• If you notice fat floating at the top of a homemade soup, stew, or sauce right before you serve it, quickly dip an ice cube into the hot liquid. Excess fat will congeal on the surface.

• To brown ground beef: Start with a cold nonstick pan. Pour browned beef into a colander or strainer. Let it drain, then turn it out into a double layer of paper towels and blot dry.

• To brown ground beef in the microwave: Put the ground beef in a

TRADITIONAL MEXICAN PIE

INGREDIENT	CALORIES
1-1/2 pounds regular ground beef, browned	262
2 onions, chopped	8
1 garlic clove, minced	0
1/4 cup oil for frying	90
2 28-ounce cans tomatoes	40
Salt and pepper to taste	0
2 (4-ounce) cans green chiles	7
12 corn tortillas	162
4 cups grated Monterey Jack cheese	455
2 cups dairy sour cream	102
1/4 cup enchilada sauce	10
	1129

LEAN MEXICAN PIE

INGREDIENT	CALORIES
1-1/2 pounds lean ground beef, browned and drained	186
2 onions, chopped	8
1 garlic clove, minced	0
2 (28-ounce) cans tomatoes	40
Salt and pepper to taste	0
2 (4-ounce) cans green chiles	7
1/4 cup enchilada sauce	10
12 corn tortillas	162
2 cups shredded part-skim Mozzarella cheese	69
1 cup Cheddar cheese	56
2 cups low-fat plain yogurt	34
	605

Sauté onions and garlic in 2 tablespoons of oil until transparent. Add tomatoes, salt, pepper and simmer for 10 minutes.

Stir in chiles. Heat about 1/2 inch of oil in a small skillet. Dip each tortilla into hot oil just to soften, about 5 seconds. Remove from oil and drain on paper towels.

In 2 (2-quart) casserole dishes, make layers of tortillas, sauce, beef and grated cheese. Repeat layers, ending with cheese. Bake uncovered at 350F for 30 minutes. Top with sour cream just before serving. Makes 8 servings.

Spray a nonstick pan with vegetable spray. Sauté onions and garlic in the pan until transparent. Add tomatoes, salt and pepper and simmer for 10 minutes.

Stir in chiles. Heat about 1/4 cup enchilada sauce in a small skillet. Dip each tortilla into hot sauce just to soften. Remove from sauce, and drain on paper towels. Add leftover enchilada sauce to tomato chili mixture.

In 2 (2-quart) casserole dishes, make layers of tortillas, sauce, beef and grated cheese. Repeat layers, ending with the cheese. Bake uncovered at 350F for 30 minutes. Top with yogurt just before serving. Makes 8 servings.

microwave-safe colander lined with paper towels. Place the colander on a glass pie plate and place in the microwave. Cook on a medium setting until the meat is brown, stopping the oven occasionally to break up the meat with a fork. Continue cooking until the meat is browned and the fat has drained into the glass dish. Discard fat and continue with the recipe.

• Substitute ground turkey for ground beef in your favorite chili recipe.

• If you use reduced-calorie products to modify your recipes, remember that not all can be automatically substituted for their less-lean counterpart. For instance diet margarine and spread products contain more water than regular butter or margarine. Generally speaking, they are best used for spreading instead of in baking goods or as a topping on popcorn.

The recipes in this book are packed with nutrition. They are low in fat and cholesterol, yet high in fiber and flavor. Although salt is kept to a minimum, these recipes are by no means salt-free. If you must restrict your sodium intake, substitute salt-free ingredients and limit the added salt. In these recipes fresh foods are recommended over processed, and the ingredients are commonly found in most grocery stores.

Each Food & Fitness recipe is analyzed by a computer program that uses the USDA Handbook 8 and 4, 5 and 6 as the data base. The nutritional information at the end of each recipe includes: total calories, grams of carbohydrate, grams of protein, grams of fat and milligrams of cholesterol per serving.

The leads of many of the recipes refer to the RDA's and US RDA'S.

RDA'S—WHAT ARE THEY?

The Recommended Dietary Allowances (RDA's) represent a measuring stick to help us evaluate our dietary intake. They tell us how much of a nutrient specific population groups should eat over time.

No two individuals have exactly the same nutritional needs. The RDA's are simply general guidelines for groups, as opposed to exact dietary recommendations for an individual. They represent average amounts of nutrients considered adequate to meet the known nutritional needs for most healthy people.

For nutrients other than energy, the RDA's include a margin of safety to account for individual variation. The RDA's are different than the minimum daily requirements (MDR's). The MDR's are the absolute least amount of a nutrient that a person needs to prevent disease. For instance, the RDA for vitamin C is 60 mg., while the MDR is 10 mg.

You probably get over and above the RDA's for most nutrients by eating a balanced diet. For example, an 8-ounce glass of orange juice provides about 160 percent of the RDA for vitamin C.

The RDA's are revised about every 5 years to keep up with the changes in scientific literature. The most current is the 1980 edition of the RDA's which is found on page 204.

US RDA'S

The United States Recommended Dietary Allowances (US RDA's) are a variation of the RDA's, and are used to evaluate the recipes in this book. The US RDA's were developed by the Food and Drug Administration (FDA) as a tool for food labeling. The nutrient breakdown on the label of a food product is based on the US RDA's. Generally speaking, they represent the highest level of the RDA (the 1968 edition) for each nutrient in each of the life cycle categories—infants, children, males and females who are not pregnant or lactating. For example, if a recipe supplies 100 percent of the US RDA for iron, it would supply the maximum 18 mg of iron recommended for women, as opposed to the 10 mg recommended for males.

Many athletes argue that they have different nutritional needs than the "average healthy person." They think the RDA's are not specific enough for them. This may be true, but research shows that the nutritional needs of an athlete are very similar to those of a person with a sedentary lifestyle. Until research shows otherwise, most nutritionists will assume that the margin of safety built into the RDA's will allow for the special nutritional needs of someone who exercises strenuously.

APPETIZERS

When it's party time, it's easy to fall off the wagon with food. Appetizers are eaten without notice, and they are usually loaded with sodium and fat. Have you ever enjoyed so many goodies before dinner that you had a less than ravenous appetite when it was time to sit down at the table?

By its definition, an appetizer is designed to stimulate the appetite, not suppress it. From a nutritional point of view, it should be packed with vitamins and minerals. For an easy-to-make appetizer that does both jobs, try Mushroom Caviar, page 54, or Dilled Tuna Mousse, page 57. If Mexican food is your style, dip a Lean Tortilla Chip, page 59, into Roasted Sweet Pepper Salsa, page 55. Shrimp Saganaki, page 60, is such a fabulous appetizer, if there are only two of you, you may want to serve it as a main entree.

Whether you call it snacking or grazing, most of us eat in bits and pieces throughout the day. Eating healthy tidbits throughout the day instead of eating just one meal a day can help stoke the body's furnace, causing more calories to be burned up. When you have a between-meal craving, reach for an apple or carrot, a few peanuts or raisins, a rice cake or pretzels to give you satisfaction. Go easy on processed snack foods that are loaded with saturated fat.

Whether you serve it in a wedge or use it as a base for a spread, cheese makes a quick and delicious appetizer. High-fat cheese is best eaten in small quantities and at special occasions. The American Heart Association recommends that a person consuming 1800 calories per day should limit his fat to a total of 60 grams. That adds up quickly when four (3/4-inch) cubes of Cheddar cheese—the size that fits neatly on a wooden pick—contain 10 grams of fat.

TO DRINK OR NOT TO DRINK

You may think appetizers and alcoholic beverages make a great team, but to serve before a meal in terms of calories, alcohol ranks as junk food since it supplies little in the way of nutritional value. When you use spirits in cooking, the alcohol evaporates. A dry table wine will lose 85% of its calories when subjected to prolonged or high heat and the alcohol evaporates. Taken as a beverage, alcohol supplies 7 calories per gram as compared to 4 calories from carbohydrates, 4 calories from protein and 9 calories from fat. It takes approximately 9 grams of alcohol to make one drink. One serving is equivalent to one jigger (1-1/2 ounces) of 80 proof distilled spirits, one (12-ounce) glass of regular beer, one (4-ounce) glass of American wine or 3 ounces of sherry.

Overnight Cheese

This tangy cheese is virtually fat-free. Use it as a spread on thinly sliced bagels, rice cakes, crisp rye crackers or combine it with your favorite seasonings for an easy vegetable dip. Read the ingredient list on the yogurt carton carefully; the yogurt will not drain if it contains gelatin.

1 pint plain low-fat yogurt without gelatin (2 cups)
1 teaspoon dried dill *or* 2 tablespoons instant minced onion
(optional)

Line the filter holder of a drip coffee pot with a coffee filter; place over coffee pot. If a drip coffee pot is not available, line a colander with a clean dish towel; set colander in a deep pan. Spoon in yogurt. Cover with plastic wrap; refrigerate 8 hours. Scoop out cheese and use at once or place in a container with a tight-fitting lid and refrigerate for up to 3 days. Serve plain or add seasoning. If using dill, stir in dill until evenly blended. Cover and refrigerate 4 hours for flavors to blend. If using onion, place onion in a small dry skillet. Cook over medium heat 30 to 60 seconds or until onion is toasted; cool. Stir onion into cheese just before serving so onion stays crunchy. Makes 1 cup cheese.

PER SERVING: 2 tablespoons

CALORIES	CARBOHYDRATES	PROTEIN	FAT	CHOLESTEROL
34	5 gm	3 gm	0 gm	1 mg

Artichoke-Chile Dip

For convenience and flavor, canned artichoke hearts packed in water and canned green chiles are two good staples to keep on hand. This dip flavorfully stretches Neufchâtel cheese to keep fat and calories at a minimum. Serve with a basket of crisp vegetables or use it as a low-fat filling for a pocket-bread sandwich.

1 (8-oz.) pkg. Neufchâtel cheese, room temperature
1/4 cup low-fat sour cream
1 (14-oz.) can water-packed artichoke hearts, drained, coarsely
**   chopped**
2 green onions with 2 inches of green tops, minced
1/4 cup canned diced green chiles
3 drops hot pepper sauce
Salt to taste

In a medium-size bowl, stir together Neufchâtel cheese and sour cream until smooth. Stir in artichokes, green onions, chiles and pepper sauce. Add salt to taste. Spoon into a serving container; cover. Refrigerate at least 2 hours for flavors to blend or for up to 2 days. Makes 2 cups.

PER SERVING: 2 tablespoons

CALORIES	CARBOHYDRATES	PROTEIN	FAT	CHOLESTEROL
46	3 gm	2 gm	3 gm	10 mg

Clam Dip

You gain protein and trim calories, fat and sodium in this streamlined version of the classic clam dip. For extra-lean snacking, serve it with a variety of vegetable dippers: red bell pepper, jicama and zucchini strips; broccoli or cauliflower flowerets; and plump red radishes.

      1 cup low-fat cottage cheese (8 oz.)
      1 (6-1/2-oz.) can chopped *or* minced clams, drained
      1 green onion, minced, including top
      2 teaspoons lemon juice
      1/2 teaspoon prepared horseradish
      3 drops hot pepper sauce

In a medium-size bowl, combine all ingredients until well mixed. Spoon into a serving container. Serve at once or cover and refrigerate for up to 2 days. Makes 1-1/4 cups.

PER SERVING: 2 tablespoons

CALORIES	CARBOHYDRATES	PROTEIN	FAT	CHOLESTEROL
35	1 gm	6 gm	1 gm	13 mg

Crunchy & Creamy Spinach Dip

This version of the popular party-pleasing spinach dip not only tastes good, but it is also good for you. For a tailgate picnic or outdoor barbecue, serve the dip in a hollowed-out, one-pound, round loaf of French bread. After removing the soft insides, cut the bread in chunks and serve in a basket as a base for the dip along with small raw mushrooms and cherry tomatoes.

      1 (10-oz.) pkg. frozen chopped spinach, thawed, drained, *or*
        1 cup cooked spinach, drained, chopped
      1/3 cup finely chopped parsley
      4 green onions, finely chopped, including tops
      1/2 cup plain low-fat yogurt
      1/2 cup commercially prepared reduced-calorie mayonnaise
      1 tablespoon lemon juice
      1/8 teaspoon ground nutmeg
      1/3 cup sliced water chestnuts, coarsely chopped
      Salt and red (cayenne) pepper to taste

With cupped hands, squeeze spinach dry; place in a medium-size bowl. Add parsley, green onions, yogurt, mayonnaise, lemon juice and nutmeg; mix well. Stir in water chestnuts. Add salt and red pepper to taste. Spoon into a serving container; cover. Refrigerate at least 2 hours for flavors to blend, or for up to 2 days. Makes 2-1/4 cups.

PER SERVING: 3 tablespoons

CALORIES	CARBOHYDRATES	PROTEIN	FAT	CHOLESTEROL
47	3 gm	1 gm	4 gm	2 mg

Eggplant Dip

This dip is deceiving because it has a creamy texture, yet is a good source of fiber. Serve it with Pocket-Bread Toasts, page 60 or crisp vegetables.

> 1 medium-size eggplant (1 lb.)
> 3 tablespoons tahini (sesame seed paste)
> 1/4 cup lemon juice
> 2 garlic cloves, pressed *or* minced
> 1/4 teaspoon ground cumin
> Salt and pepper to taste
> 2 tablespoons chopped parsley

Preheat oven to 400F (205C). Pierce unpeeled eggplant in several places with a fork to allow steam to escape when baked. Place in a pie pan. Bake 50 minutes or until fork-tender; cool. Peel off skin; cut off stem. Finely chop eggplant. Place in a colander for 30 minutes to drain. In a medium-size bowl, combine tahini, lemon juice, garlic, and cumin; stir until smooth. Add eggplant; stir until well mixed. Add salt and pepper to taste. Let stand at least 30 minutes for flavors to blend, or cover and refrigerate for up to 2 days. If refrigerated, bring to room temperature before serving. To serve, place in a serving bowl; sprinkle with parsley. Makes 1-2/3 cups.

PER SERVING: 3 tablespoons

CALORIES	CARBOHYDRATES	PROTEIN	FAT	CHOLESTEROL
25	3 gm	1 gm	1 gm	0 mg

Guacamole

Whoever nicknamed guacamole "poor man's butter" may not have realized how lucky a poor man can be. Avocado, the base of guacamole, is rich in fat. Because of the avocado's built-in richness, you don't need to add extra fat to make this creamy spread. It is delicious served with Lean Tortilla Chips, page 59, or as a topping for burritos, tostados or Taco Salad, page 160.

> 2 large ripe avocados (1 lb. *total*)
> 2 tablespoons lemon *or* lime juice
> 1 small tomato, finely chopped (1/2 cup)
> 2 tablespoons minced onion
> 2 or 3 canned green chiles, seeded, diced
> 2 tablespoons chopped cilantro leaves
> Salt to taste

Halve avocados lengthwise; remove pits. With a spoon, scoop pulp from shells into a small bowl. Mash with a fork. Stir in lemon juice, tomato, onion, chiles and cilantro; mix lightly. Salt to taste. Spoon into a serving container. Serve at once or cover and refrigerate for up to 2 hours. Makes 2 cups.

PER SERVING: 2 tablespoons

CALORIES	CARBOHYDRATES	PROTEIN	FAT	CHOLESTEROL
131	7 gm	2 gm	12 gm	0 mg

Curry Dip

Cherry tomatoes and blanched asparagus spears make perfect partners for this spicy dip. Steam or boil the asparagus until crisp-tender, chill briefly in ice water, then pat dry with paper towels before serving.

> 1/2 cup low-fat sour cream (4 oz.)
> 2 tablespoons lemon juice
> 1 teaspoon curry powder

In a small bowl, whisk together all ingredients until smooth. Transfer to a serving bowl; cover. Refrigerate at least 30 minutes for flavors to blend or for up to 3 days. Makes 1/2 cup.

PER SERVING: 1 tablespoon

CALORIES	CARBOHYDRATES	PROTEIN	FAT	CHOLESTEROL
10	1 gm	1 gm	1 gm	1 mg

Mushroom Caviar

This caviar is inexpensive enough to serve anytime, not just on special occasions. Sweet and creamy, it tastes terrific spread on rye cocktail rounds, lavosh or just about any type of unbuttered, unsalted crisp cracker.

> 1/2 lb. mushrooms
> 1 tablespoon olive oil
> 1 small onion, finely chopped (2/3 cup)
> 2 tablespoons chopped parsley
> 1/4 teaspoon dried thyme
> 3 tablespoons dry white wine
> 1/4 cup low-fat sour cream
> Salt and pepper to taste
> Paprika

In a food processor, process mushrooms until finely but evenly chopped; scrape down sides of bowl if necessary. If a food processor is not available, finely chop mushrooms with a knife. In a large skillet heat oil over medium heat. Add onion; cook until soft but not browned. Add mushrooms, parsley, thyme and wine. Increase heat to medium-high. Cook 6 to 8 minutes or until liquid evaporates and mixture is dark brown. Remove from heat; cool. Stir in sour cream and salt and pepper to taste, then spoon into a serving container. Sprinkle lightly with paprika. Serve or cover and refrigerate for up to 2 days. Makes 1 cup.

PER SERVING: 1 tablespoon

CALORIES	CARBOHYDRATES	PROTEIN	FAT	CHOLESTEROL
10	1 gm	0 gm	1 gm	0 mg

Roasted Sweet Pepper Salsa

What a tasty way to get your vitamin C and vitamin A. In this mildly hot salsa, red bell peppers and tomatoes supply generous amounts of both vitamins. Scoop up the salsa with low-fat chips for an appetizer or serve it alongside grilled meat, fish or poultry as a flavor accent.

> 2 large red bell peppers (3/4 lb. *total*)
> 3 fresh *or* canned tomatillos
> 4 medium-size tomatoes, peeled, seeded, coarsely chopped
>   (1 lb. *total*)
> 2 small fresh Serrano *or* jalapeno chiles, seeded, finely
>   chopped
> 1 small onion, chopped (2/3 cup)
> 2 tablespoons chopped cilantro leaves
> 2 tablespoons lime juice
> 1 tablespoon olive oil
> 1/2 teaspoon ground cumin
> Salt to taste

Preheat broiler. Put whole bell peppers in a shallow ovenproof pan; place 1 inch under preheated broiler. Broil, turning frequently with tongs, until peppers are blistered and charred on all sides. Place peppers in a plastic bag; close bag tightly. Let peppers sweat 15 minutes to loosen skins. Remove peppers from bag and peel; discard skins, seeds and pith. Coarsely chop peppers; place in a large bowl. Remove papery husks from fresh tomatillos; wash and coarsely chop. (If using canned tomatillos, drain and coarsely chop.) Add tomatillos to bell peppers along with tomatoes, chiles, onion, cilantro, lime juice, olive oil and cumin; mix well. Add salt to taste; cover. Refrigerate at least 1 hour for flavors to blend, or for up to 5 days. Makes 3 cups.

PER SERVING: 1/4 cup

CALORIES	CARBOHYDRATES	PROTEIN	FAT	CHOLESTEROL
35	6 gm	1 gm	1.5 gm	0 mg

Ten-Minute Salsa

When vine-ripened tomatoes are out-of-season, make this zingy, chunky salsa from canned tomatoes. Serve over omelets or alongside hamburgers or fish.

2 (16-oz. *each*) cans whole peeled tomatoes, drained, coarsely
   chopped
1 (4-oz.) can diced green chiles
1 cup finely chopped green onions, including tops (about 6)
2 teaspoons red wine vinegar
1/2 teaspoon dried oregano
1 teaspoon vegetable oil
Salt to taste

In a container with a tight-fitting lid, combine tomatoes, chiles, green onions, wine vinegar, oregano and oil; stir to blend. Add salt to taste; stir until well mixed. Serve at once or cover and refrigerate for up to 5 days. Makes 3-1/4 cups.

PER SERVING: 1/4 cup				
CALORIES	CARBOHYDRATES	PROTEIN	FAT	CHOLESTEROL
22	4 gm	1 gm	.5 gm	0 mg

Caponata

To replace potassium after a long run, here's a good summertime snack. One serving has about three times more potassium than is in one cup of orange juice. Serve it on crackers, wrap up a spoonful in a lettuce leaf, or tuck it inside half a pocket bread for a great sandwich.

2 tablespoons olive oil
1 medium-size eggplant, unpeeled, cut in 3/4-inch cubes (1 lb.)
1 cup water
1 medium-size onion, chopped (5 oz.)
3 large celery stalks, sliced
1/4 cup tomato paste
1/4 cup red wine vinegar
1 tablespoon sugar
1 tablespoon capers, rinsed, drained
Salt and pepper to taste

In a wide nonstick skillet or 5-quart saucepan that has a lid heat oil over medium heat. Add eggplant and 1/4 cup of the water. Cover; cook 5 minutes. Uncover; cook 5 minutes longer or until liquid evaporates and eggplant just begins to brown. Stir in onion and celery; cook, uncovered, until onion is soft but not browned. In a small bowl, whisk together tomato paste, wine vinegar, sugar and the remaining 3/4 cup water. Add capers. Stir mixture into eggplant. Cover; simmer 10 minutes. Uncover; cook 10 minutes longer or until eggplant is tender and mixture thickens. Add salt and pepper to taste. Remove from heat and let cool. Spoon into a serving container; serve at once, or cool, cover and refrigerate for up to 4 days. Serve cold or at room temperature. Makes 4 cups.

PER SERVING: 1/4 cup				
CALORIES	CARBOHYDRATES	PROTEIN	FAT	CHOLESTEROL
151	18 gm	4 gm	7 gm	0 mg

Dilled Tuna Mousse

Who ever heard of a low-fat party food? This is it. One tablespoon of this recipe is virtually fat-free, yet is loaded with several vitamins and minerals like thiamin, riboflavin, niacin and iron. For an elegant first course, line plates with butter lettuce leaves and place 3 tablespoons Dilled Tuna Mousse on each.

> 1 (1/4-oz.) envelope unflavored gelatin (about 1 tablespoon)
> 1/4 cup cold water
> 3/4 cup spicy vegetable juice cocktail
> 1/2 cup plain low-fat yogurt
> 1/2 cup low-fat sour cream
> 1 teaspoon dried dill
> 1/4 teaspoon salt
> 1 (6-1/2-oz.) can water-pack tuna, drained, flaked
> 2 teaspoons capers, rinsed, drained, chopped
> 2 parsley sprigs
> 1 lb. 28-inch long baguette, cut in 48 thin slices

In a small bowl, stir gelatin into cold water; let stand 3 minutes to soften. In a small pan, bring vegetable juice cocktail to a simmer over medium heat. Add gelatin; stir until gelatin is dissolved. Remove from heat; cool to room temperature. In a medium-size bowl, combine yogurt, sour cream, dill, salt and gelatin mixture. Beat until well blended. Place bowl into a large bowl filled with ice water; stir occasionally until mixture mounds slightly when dropped from a spoon, about 25 minutes. Remove bowl from ice water. Stir in tuna and capers. Grease a 2-1/2- to 3-cup mold with vegetable nonstick cooking spray. Spoon tuna mixture into mold. Cover and refrigerate until firm, at least 4 hours or for up to 2 days. To serve, unmold onto a plate. Garnish with parsley sprigs. To serve, spread 1 tablespoon of mousse on 1 baguette slice. Makes 2-1/2 cups.

PER SERVING: 1 tablespoon				
CALORIES	CARBOHYDRATES	PROTEIN	FAT	CHOLESTEROL
44	7 gm	3 gm	1 gm	3 mg

Skagway Salmon

For an appetizer big on flavor, pickled salmon is an inexpensive and delicious alternative to lox. It is high in protein, low in fat and has less salt than two bread slices. Eaten with your hands, it can be messy, so be sure to have plenty of napkins available.

> **1 teaspoon salt**
> **1 lb. salmon steaks** *or* **fillet, boned, skinned**
> **1-1/2 cups water**
> **1/2 cup distilled white vinegar**
> **1/4 cup sugar**
> **1/2 bay leaf**
> **1 piece cinnamon stick (2 inches)**
> **1 quarter-size slice fresh gingerroot, crushed with knife blade**
> **1/2 lemon, sliced**
> **1 medium-size onion, thinly sliced (5 oz.)**

Rub salt into fish covering all sides; place in a medium-size bowl. Cover; refrigerate at least 1 hour. Rinse fish thoroughly in cold water; drain. In a 2-quart saucepan, combine water, vinegar, sugar, bay leaf, cinnamon stick, ginger and lemon. Bring to a boil over high heat; reduce heat. Simmer 5 minutes. Add fish; simmer, uncovered, 4 minutes or until fish just begins to turn opaque (Fish will complete cooking as it cools in the pickling broth.) Separate onion into rings; place in a 1-quart container with a tight-fitting lid. Pour fish and pickling liquid over onion; cool. Cover and refrigerate at least 4 hours or for up to 3 days. To serve, lift fish and onion rings from pickling mixture with a slotted spoon; discard liquid. Break fish into bite-size pieces. Arrange fish on platter with onion rings. Makes 8 appetizer servings.

PER SERVING: 1/8 of total recipe				
CALORIES	CARBOHYDRATES	PROTEIN	FAT	CHOLESTEROL
122	5 gm	15 gm	4 gm	26 mg

Marinated Mushrooms

You may want to double this recipe. These flavorful mushrooms are handy to have on hand for impromptu entertaining, between-meal snacking and bag or briefcase lunches.

> 24 medium-size mushrooms (1/2 lb.)
> 2 tablespoons red wine vinegar
> 2 teaspoons olive oil
> 1/4 teaspoon salt
> 1/4 teaspoon dried oregano
> 1/4 teaspoon dried rosemary, crumbled
> 1 tablespoon chopped parsley
> Pepper to taste
> 1 small garlic clove

In a 2-quart saucepan bring 2 cups water to a rapid boil over high heat. Add mushrooms; cover, reduce heat. Simmer 10 minutes or until mushrooms are just barely fork-tender; drain. In a container with a tight-fitting lid, combine mushrooms, wine vinegar, oil, salt, oregano, rosemary and parsley. Add pepper to taste. Stick garlic on a wooden pick; add to mushrooms. Cover, and refrigerate at least 4 hours or for up to 4 days. Discard garlic after 4 hours unless you prefer a stronger garlic flavor. Makes 4 servings.

PER SERVING: 6 mushrooms

CALORIES	CARBOHYDRATES	PROTEIN	FAT	CHOLESTEROL
31	2 gm	1 gm	2 gm	0 mg

Lean Tortilla Chips

Compared to the same amount of commercially prepared corn tortilla chips, this low-fat version, made with flour tortillas, has about the same number of calories, but only one-fourth the amount of fat. For an easy hors d'oeuvre, serve chips with Ten-Minute Salsa, page 56, or Roasted Sweet Pepper Salsa, page 55.

> 4 (8-inch) whole-wheat flour tortillas
> 4 (8-inch) regular flour tortillas
> Cold water

Preheat oven to 350F (175C). One at a time, quickly *dip* each tortilla in bowl of cold water; drain. Cut each tortilla into 8 triangles. Place triangles, in a single layer, in 2 large baking pans. Place one pan in preheated oven and bake 10 minutes or until chips are crisp and just begin to lightly brown; remove from oven and cool. Repeat with remaining pan. Store in an airtight container for up to 5 days. Makes 64 chips.

PER SERVING: 6 chips

CALORIES	CARBOHYDRATES	PROTEIN	FAT	CHOLESTEROL
70	13 gm	2 gm	1 gm	0.5 mg

Pocket-Bread Toasts

Here is a fat-free chip to serve with a dip, a salsa or a spread. Whole-wheat pocket bread is not as widely available as pocket bread made with white flour, but it is worth looking for if you like the nut-like sweetness of whole-wheat.

4 (6-inch) whole-wheat pocket breads
4 (6-inch) regular pocket breads

Preheat oven to 350F (175C). Cut around pocket bread edges to make 2 flat rounds from each bread. Cut each round in 6 triangles. Place triangles, in a single layer, in 2 large baking pans. Place one pan in preheated oven and bake 5 minutes. Turn triangles over. Continue to bake 5 minutes longer or until lightly toasted; cool. Repeat with remaining pan. Store in an airtight container up to 5 days. Makes 96 toast triangles.

PER SERVING: 6 triangles

CALORIES	CARBOHYDRATES	PROTEIN	FAT	CHOLESTEROL
54	11 gm	2 gm	0.5 gm	trace

Shrimp Saganaki

Once you begin to eat this specialty of Greek travernas you may want to make a meal of it. As an appetizer, offer wooden skewers so each person can spear an assortment of these low-fat goodies. As an entree, serve the lemony combination of shrimp and vegetables over steamed rice. If you serve this as an entree with rice for 3 you count 211 calories, 14 grams carbohydrates, 14 grams protein, 11 grams fat and 84 milligrams cholesterol per serving.

2 tablespoons olive oil
2 large garlic cloves, pressed *or* minced
1/2 lb. medium-size raw shrimp, shelled, deveined
1/4 lb. medium-size mushrooms, cut in half lengthwise
1 (14-oz.) can artichoke hearts packed in water, drained,
**   cut in half**
1/2 teaspoon dried oregano
1/2 teaspoon dried dill
2 tablespoons lemon juice
2 tablespoons chopped parsley
Pepper to taste

In a large skillet heat oil over medium-high heat. Add garlic; cook 30 seconds. Add shrimp and mushrooms; cook 3 minutes or just until shrimp start to turn pink. Add artichoke hearts, oregano and dill; cook 1 minute. Add lemon juice and parsley; cook 2 minutes to blend flavors. Add pepper to taste. Spoon into a serving bowl and serve hot. Provide wooden skewers for spearing. Makes 8 appetizer servings.

PER APPETIZER SERVING: 1/8 of total recipe

CALORIES	CARBOHYDRATES	PROTEIN	FAT	CHOLESTEROL
64	5 gm	5 gm	4 gm	31 mg

Sesame Wine Chicken

It's nice to know that an appetizer that tastes so good is good for you too. One serving supplies 42% of the US RDA for protein and 46% of the US RDA for niacin. If you have leftover chicken, pack it in a lunch or use the shreds to garnish a spinach salad.

1 lb. chicken breasts, skin removed
1-1/2 cups water
1 green onion, cut in half
1 quarter-size slice fresh gingerroot, crushed with knife blade
1/2 teaspoon salt
1/2 teaspoon sugar
1/2 cup dry white wine
1/2 teaspoon sesame oil
2 green lettuce leaves
1 teaspoon sesame seeds

In a saucepan, combine chicken breasts, water, green onion, ginger, salt and sugar. Heat to simmering over medium heat. Cover; simmer 20 minutes. Remove chicken from broth; let stand until cool enough to handle. Strain broth. Return broth to clean pan; cook, uncovered, over medium heat until reduced to 1/2 cup; cool. Pull chicken off bones; shred into bite-size pieces. Place chicken in a plastic bag. Add cooled broth, wine and sesame oil. Seal bag; turn bag over to distribute marinade. Refrigerate at least 1 day or for up to 3 days; turn bag occasionally to distribute marinade. To serve, drain chicken. Arrange lettuce leaves on a serving plate; place chicken on top of lettuce. Place sesame seeds in a dry skillet. Toast over low heat, shaking skillet frequently, for 2 minutes or until seeds turn golden and begin to pop. Sprinkle over chicken. Provide wooden picks for spearing. Makes 6 appetizer servings.

PER SERVING: 1/6 of total recipe

CALORIES	CARBOHYDRATES	PROTEIN	FAT	CHOLESTEROL
82	1 gm	15 gm	2 gm	43 mg

SOUPS

The magic of soup is that it offers so much in satisfaction, flavor and nutritional value and adds so little in calories from fat. It is the perfect fitness food both in winter and summer. In this chapter there is a selection of nutrient-dense soups for every occasion.

Making soup from scratch is not short order cooking. Soups made with dried beans or legumes take time. They are a good choice for weekend cooking because these soups require little attention while they slowly simmer. Once cooked, they become convenient one-dish meals. Cool the soup, then package in meal-size portions, in plastic seal bags, and freeze for later use. Just heat the quantity you want for a quick lunch or dinner.

Soups made without dried beans and legumes go together so quickly that it makes sense to prepare them in smaller quantities. You'll find choices for soup to accompany a salad or sandwich as well as soups hearty enough to make a meal-in-a-bowl.

WHICH STOCK IS BEST?

On a rating of one to three, homemade chicken broth ranks as first choice for soup stock if you want total control of the fat and sodium content. For convenience and flavor, these recipes call for ready-to-use (regular-strength) canned chicken broth which is less salty than stock made from cubes or granules of chicken stock base. If you are very concerned about your sodium intake make soups with low-sodium chicken bouillon granules. When making soup with canned chicken broth, do not add salt until the end of cooking. Taste, and you may find extra salt is not necessary. If you wish to reduce the sodium content even more without sacrificing flavor, dilute the canned broth with an equal amount of water. For fat-free canned chicken broth, remove the lid, rather than punching a hole in the top of the can, and discard the bit of fat which floats on the surface.

CUPS VERSUS POUNDS

Unlike many recipes, the proportions in soup making are not critical. If you have one stalk of celery and the recipe calls for two, or if you use a medium-size carrot when the recipe calls for a large one, the results will still taste good. Because it is faster to dice a small potato and add it to the kettle rather than to dice a potato, measure out 1 cup, then add it to the kettle, we have, when it was appropriate, listed fruits and vegetables by size. The pounds or ounces we have used are those used to calculate the nutritional data and will also serve as your shopping guide. You may consider a large zucchini to be 6 inches long while the home gardener thinks a zucchini large when it reaches 12 inches in length.

Sonora-Style Bean Soup

Dried beans are a great source of fiber and here is a tasty way to include them in your diet. To make a more complete protein soup, place 1/4 cup cooked rice in each bowl before ladling in the soup.

> 1 tablespoon vegetable oil
> 1 small onion, chopped (3 oz.)
> 1 garlic clove, pressed *or* minced
> 1 large celery stalk, cut in half lengthwise, thinly sliced
> 2 tablespoons canned diced green chiles
> 1/4 teaspoon ground cumin
> 1/4 teaspoon dried oregano
> 2 (14-1/2-oz. *each*) cans regular-strength chicken broth *or*
>   3-1/2 cups homemade chicken broth
> 1 tablespoon tomato paste
> 3 cups cooked pinto beans *or* 1 (1 lb. 14-oz.) can
>   pinto beans, drained
> 1 cup water
> Salt to taste
> 1/3 cup shredded Cheddar cheese (1-1/2 oz.)
> 2 tablespoons chopped cilantro leaves

In a 3-quart saucepan heat oil over medium heat. Add onion, garlic and celery; cook until onion is soft but not browned. Add chiles, cumin and oregano; cook for 1 minute. Add chicken broth, tomato paste and 1-1/2 cups of the beans. In a blender or food processor, combine the remaining 1-1/2 cups beans and water; process until smooth. Add to soup. Bring to a boil over high heat; reduce heat. Cover; simmer 15 minutes. Add salt to taste. Ladle hot soup into individual bowls. Garnish each serving with cheese and cilantro. Makes 4 (1-1/2-cup) servings.

PER SERVING: 1-1/2 cups

CALORIES	CARBOHYDRATES	PROTEIN	FAT	CHOLESTEROL
279	35 gm	18 gm	9 gm	9 mg

Saving Leftover Tomato Paste:
After opening the tomato paste, spoon the leftover portion, in 1-tablespoon amounts, on a pie plate, then freeze. When frozen, transfer to a plastic bag, seal and return to the freezer.

Split Pea Soup with Kale

A hearty "main-dish" soup, yet it is low in fat. One serving provides 43% of the US RDA for protein, yet has less fat than one tablespoon of cream cheese. This soup also contains a significant amount of iron. One serving provides almost 1/4 of the US RDA for this important energy-related mineral.

> **1 cup dried split peas, rinsed (5 oz.)**
> **1 lb. center-cut beef shank**
> **1/2 medium-size sweet potato, peeled, diced (4 oz.)**
> **1 large potato, peeled, diced (8 oz.)**
> **12 cups water**
> **2 medium-size potatoes (12 oz. *total*)**
> **1 bunch kale *or* mustard greens, including stems (12 oz.)**
> **Salt to taste**

In a 5-quart kettle, combine split peas, beef shank, sweet potato, diced potato and water. Bring to a boil over high heat; reduce heat. Cover; simmer 2 hours or until peas are very tender. With a slotted spoon, remove meat to a plate. In a blender, process split pea-potato mixture, a portion at a time, until smooth. Return to kettle. Cut meat into bite-size pieces, discarding bone and gristle. Return meat to kettle. Peel potatoes; cut in 1-1/2-inch cubes and add to soup. Heat soup to simmering; cover and simmer 15 minutes. Coarsely chop kale; add to soup. Cover; simmer 10 minutes or until potatoes are tender. Add salt to taste. Serve in individual bowls. Makes 8 (1-1/3-cup) servings.

PER SERVING: 1-1/3 cups

CALORIES	CARBOHYDRATES	PROTEIN	FAT	CHOLESTEROL
245	35 gm	19 gm	4 gm	29 mg

Guatemalan Black Bean Soup

Latin American flavors spice this hearty soup. One serving provides 50% of the US RDA for protein, yet contains less fat than 4 large black olives.

> **1 lb. dried black beans**
> **1 lb. ham shank, cut in 3 pieces, fat trimmed**
> **1 medium-size onion, chopped (5 oz.)**
> **2 large celery stalks with leaves, chopped**
> **2 garlic cloves, pressed *or* minced**
> **1 bay leaf**
> **1/2 teaspoon dried oregano**
> **1/2 teaspoon dried basil**
> **1/2 cup dry red wine**
> **1 (8-oz.) can tomato sauce**
> **Salt to taste**
> **2 lemons, cut in wedges**

Sort beans, discarding any foreign material. Place beans in a large kettle. Add enough hot water to cover beans by 2 inches. Cover; bring to a boil over high heat; boil 2 minutes. Remove from heat and let soak, covered, for 1 hour; drain. Add 10 cups hot water, ham shank, onion, celery, garlic, bay leaf, oregano and basil. Cover with lid ajar; simmer gently for 1-1/2 hours. Add wine and tomato sauce. Continue to simmer 1 hour or until beans are very tender. With a slotted spoon, remove meat to a plate. Discard bay leaf. In a food processor or blender, process half of the beans and a little of the broth until smooth; return puree to kettle. Cut meat into bite-size pieces, discarding bone. Return meat to kettle. Heat to simmering. Add salt to taste. Pour into a tureen or serve in individual bowls. Pass lemon wedges at the table. Makes 8 (1-1/3-cup) servings.

PER SERVING: 1-1/3 cups

CALORIES	CARBOHYDRATES	PROTEIN	FAT	CHOLESTEROL
326	35 gm	30 gm	6 gm	52 mg

Tomato Lentil Soup

This low-calorie soup contains no cholesterol and only 3 grams of fat per serving. It is a great accompaniment to a broiled chicken or fish entree or a "main-dish" salad.

> **1 tablespoon olive oil**
> **1 medium-size red onion, chopped (5 oz.)**
> **2 garlic cloves, pressed *or* minced**
> **1 large celery stalk with leaves, finely chopped**
> **1/4 cup chopped green bell pepper**
> **1/4 cup dry red wine**
> **1 (16-oz.) can whole peeled tomatoes**
> **3/4 cup dried lentils, rinsed**
> **1 (14-1/2-oz.) can regular-strength chicken broth *or***
>   **1-3/4 cups homemade chicken broth**
> **1-3/4 cups water**
> **1 bay leaf**
> **1/2 teaspoon dried thyme**
> **1/2 teaspoon dried basil**
> **Salt and pepper to taste**

In a 3-quart saucepan heat oil over medium heat. Add onion, garlic, celery, and bell pepper; cook until onion is soft but not browned. Add wine; simmer for 2 minutes. Pour tomatoes and their liquid into pan. Coarsely cut up tomatoes. Add lentils, broth, water, bay leaf, thyme and basil. Bring to a boil over high heat; reduce heat. Cover; simmer 45 minutes or until lentils are tender. Remove bay leaf. Add salt and pepper to taste. Ladle hot soup into individual bowls. Makes 6 (1-cup) servings.

PER SERVING: 1 cup

CALORIES	CARBOHYDRATES	PROTEIN	FAT	CHOLESTEROL
105	14 gm	4 gm	3 gm	0 mg

Lentil & Spinach Soup

Great for lunch after a hard game of squash or racquetball, this legume combination replaces depleted potassium and stored carbohydrates. Sixty-seven percent of the total calories come from complex carbohydrates, and 1 cup supplies 2-1/2 times more potassium than 5 small oranges. An excellent "cancer-protective" food, since one serving supplies almost 100% of the US RDA for both vitamins A and C.

1-1/2 cups dried lentils, rinsed
7 cups homemade chicken broth *or* 1 (49-1/2-oz.) can
   regular-strength chicken broth and 1 cup water
1 medium-size onion, chopped (5 oz.)
2 garlic cloves, pressed *or* minced
2 medium-size thin-skinned potatoes, peeled, diced
   (10 oz. *total*)
1 bunch spinach, washed, drained, stems removed,
   coarsely chopped (12 oz.)
3 tablespoon lemon juice
Salt and freshly ground black pepper to taste
1/2 cup plain low-fat yogurt

In a 5-quart kettle, combine lentils, chicken broth, onion and garlic. Bring to a boil over high heat; reduce heat. Cover; simmer 20 minutes. Add potatoes. Cover; simmer 20 more minutes or until lentils and potatoes are tender. Stir in spinach. Cover; simmer 5 minutes longer. Add lemon juice. Add salt and pepper to taste. Ladle hot soup into individual bowls. Top each serving with 1 tablespoon yogurt. Makes 8 (1-cup) servings.

PER SERVING: 1 cup				
CALORIES	CARBOHYDRATES	PROTEIN	FAT	CHOLESTEROL
208	34 gm	15 gm	2 gm	0 mg

Curried Squash Soup

This soup is very deceiving. It is thick and satisfying, yet very low in calories and fat. One serving contains only 109 calories, has less fat than a tablespoon of salad dressing and is cholesterol-free.

1 tablespoon margarine
1 medium-size onion, chopped (5 oz.)
4 cups peeled, diced butternut squash (*about* 2 lbs.)
1 large apple, Granny Smith or Golden Delicious, cored,
   peeled, diced (8 oz.)
1 (49-1/2-oz.) can regular-strength chicken broth *or*
   6 cups homemade chicken broth
1/4 teaspoon ground nutmeg
1/4 teaspoon ground ginger
1-1/2 teaspoons curry powder
1/2 bay leaf
Dash white pepper
3 tablespoons chopped parsley

In a 3-quart saucepan melt margarine over medium heat. Add onion; cook until onion is soft but not browned. Add squash, apple, chicken broth, nutmeg, ginger, curry power, bay leaf and pepper. Bring to a boil over high heat; reduce heat. Cover; simmer 25 minutes or until squash is tender. Remove bay leaf. In a blender or food processor, process soup, a portion at a time, until very smooth. Return to pan. Heat to simmering. Serve in mugs or individual bowls. Sprinkle parsley over each serving. Makes 8 (1-cup) servings.

PER SERVING: 1 cup				
CALORIES	CARBOHYDRATES	PROTEIN	FAT	CHOLESTEROL
109	17 gm	5 gm	3 gm	0 mg

Crab & Artichoke Bisque

One cup of this soup provides about 50% of the US RDA for vitamin B_{12}, which is one nutrient often lacking when meat is excluded from the diet. Team this soup with a tossed green salad and whole-wheat bread.

> 1 (14-oz.) can artichoke hearts packed in water, drained
> 3 cups canned regular-strength chicken broth *or*
>   3 cups homemade chicken broth
> 3 tablespoons margarine
> 6 tablespoons all-purpose flour
> 2 tablespoons dry sherry
> 2 cups low-fat milk
> 1/4 teaspoon ground nutmeg
> 1/4 teaspoon paprika
> 4 drops hot pepper sauce
> 1/3 lb. crabmeat *or* surimi-style (imitation) crabmeat
> Salt to taste
> 1 tablespoon chopped fresh dill *or* 1 teaspoon dried dill

Place half the artichoke hearts and chicken broth in a blender; process until smooth. Cut remaining artichoke hearts into quarters; reserve. In a 3-quart saucepan melt margarine over medium heat. Stir in flour; cook 1 minute or until bubbly. Remove pan from heat. Gradually whisk in artichoke heart-chicken broth mixture. Add sherry. Return pan to heat. Cook, stirring, until soup comes to a boil and thickens slightly. Add milk, nutmeg, paprika, hot pepper sauce, crab and reserved artichoke hearts. Add salt to taste. Heat to simmering. Serve soup in individual bowls. Garnish each serving with dill. Makes 6 (1-cup) servings.

PER SERVING: 1 cup				
CALORIES	CARBOHYDRATES	PROTEIN	FAT	CHOLESTEROL
180	15 gm	12 gm	9 gm	32 mg

Chunky Vegetable Soup

One cup of this soup provides 50% of the US RDA for vitamin A and 63% of the US RDA for vitamin C. A good "cancer protective" food, this soup is a great pre- or post-race dish, since over half the calories are in the form of complex carbohydrates.

2 tablespoons margarine
1 medium-size onion, chopped (5 oz.)
2 celery stalks, thinly sliced
1 medium-size carrot, thinly sliced (4 oz.)
1 (16-oz.) can whole peeled tomatoes
2 cups thinly sliced cabbage
2 (14-1/2-oz. *each*) cans regular-strength chicken broth *or*
    3-1/2 cups homemade chicken broth
2 cups water
1 teaspoon dried basil
1/2 teaspoon dried oregano
2 medium-size zucchini, thinly sliced (12 oz. *total*)
1 cup medium-size pasta shells *or* corkscrew-shaped pasta
2 tablespoons chopped parsley
1 cup frozen green peas, thawed
Salt to taste
3 tablespoons grated Parmesan cheese

In a 3-quart saucepan melt margarine over medium heat. Add onion, celery, and carrot; cook until onion is soft but not browned. Pour tomatoes and their liquid into pan; coarsely cut up tomatoes. Add cabbage, chicken broth, water, basil and oregano. Bring to a boil over high heat; reduce heat. Cover; simmer 30 minutes. Increase heat so soup boils gently. Add zucchini, pasta and parsley. Cover and cook 5 minutes. Add peas. Cook 5 minutes longer or until pasta is tender but firm to the bite. Add salt to taste. Serve in individual bowls. Sprinkle 1 teaspoon Parmesan cheese over each serving. Makes 9 (1-cup) servings.

PER SERVING: 1 cup

CALORIES	CARBOHYDRATES	PROTEIN	FAT	CHOLESTEROL
145	20 gm	7 gm	4 gm	2 mg

Cool Cucumber-Dill Soup

Tangy cucumber soup is a good thirst quencher after a long day of waterskiing. This cool, refreshing soup is virtually fat-free, and one serving supplies 25% of the US RDA for vitamin C.

2 cups buttermilk
1 cup plain lowfat yogurt (8 oz.)
2 tablespoons lemon juice
2 medium-size cucumbers, peeled (1 lb. *total*)
1/4 cup chopped parsley
3 green onions, thinly sliced, including tops
1 tablespoon chopped fresh dill *or* 1 teaspoon dried dill
Salt and freshly ground black pepper to taste
6 fresh dill sprigs *or* 6 radishes, shredded (optional)

Pour buttermilk into a large bowl. Whisk in yogurt and lemon juice until smooth; set aside. Cut cucumbers in half lengthwise. Scoop out and discard seeds. Shred cucumbers or finely chop. Stir gently into buttermilk mixture along with parsley, green onions and chopped dill. Season to taste with salt and pepper. Pour into a 2-quart container with a tight-fitting lid. Cover and refrigerate at least 4 hours or for up to 3 days. Serve cold in mugs or individual bowls. Garnish each serving with a dill sprig or shredded radish if desired. Makes 6 (3/4-cup) servings.

PER SERVING: 3/4 cup				
CALORIES	CARBOHYDRATES	PROTEIN	FAT	CHOLESTEROL
70	10 gm	5 gm	0.8 gm	3 mg

Blender Gazpacho

Here's a refreshing appetizer or light lunch after a "hot" game of tennis. It's another good "cancer protective" food, supplying 50% of the US RDA for vitamin A and over 100% of the US RDA for vitamin C.

> 5 medium-size tomatoes, peeled, cored, quartered,
> (1-1/4 lbs. *total*) *or* 1 (16-oz.) can whole peeled tomatoes
> 1 medium-size cucumber, peeled, seeded, sliced (8 oz.)
> 1 medium-size onion, sliced (5 oz.)
> 3 parsley sprigs
> 1/2 teaspoon paprika
> 1/8 teaspoon ground cumin
> Dash red (cayenne) pepper
> 1 tablespoon olive oil
> 1 tablespoon red wine vinegar
> Salt to taste
> 1 green onion
> Ice cubes

In a 2-quart saucepan, combine tomatoes, cucumber, onion, parsley, paprika, cumin and red pepper. Bring to a boil over high heat; reduce heat. Cover; simmer 25 minutes or until vegetables are tender. In a blender, process soup to make a rough puree. Pour into a medium-size container with a tight-fitting lid; let cool uncovered. Stir in oil, wine vinegar and salt to taste. Cover and refrigerate at least 4 hours or for as long as 3 days. Just before serving, thinly slice green onion, including top; place one or two ice cubes in each bowl. Ladle cold soup over ice cubes. Garnish each serving with green onion. Makes 4 (3/4-cup) servings.

PER SERVING: 3/4 cup				
CALORIES	CARBOHYDRATES	PROTEIN	FAT	CHOLESTEROL
89	13 gm	4 gm	4 gm	0 mg

Broccoli Buttermilk Soup

After a long, hard bike ride, this is a great dish to replace depleted potassium and replenish muscle glycogen. One serving supplies about 1-1/2 times more potassium than is in 1 cup of orange juice. Over half the calories in this soup come from complex carbohydrates, and one serving has less fat than a teaspoon of margarine.

> 1 tablespoon margarine
> 1 medium-size onion, chopped (5 oz.)
> 1 garlic clove, pressed *or* minced
> 4 cups coarsely chopped broccoli flowerets and sliced,
>   peeled stems (1 lb.)
> 2 small potatoes, peeled, diced (8 oz. *total*)
> 2 (14-1/2-oz. *each*) cans regular-strength chicken broth *or*
>   3-1/2 cups homemade chicken broth
> 1/2 teaspoon dried basil
> 2 cups buttermilk
> 1/8 teaspoon ground nutmeg
> Dash red (cayenne) pepper

In a 3-quart saucepan melt margarine over medium heat. Add onion and garlic; cook until onion is soft but not browned. Add broccoli, potatoes, chicken broth and basil. Bring to a boil over high heat; reduce heat. Cover; simmer 30 minutes or until vegetables are tender. In a blender or food processor, process soup, a portion at a time, until very smooth. Return to pan. Whisk in buttermilk, nutmeg and red pepper. Heat to simmering. Serve in mugs or bowls. Makes 7 (1-cup) servings.

PER SERVING: 1 cup				
CALORIES	CARBOHYDRATES	PROTEIN	FAT	CHOLESTEROL
120	15 gm	8 gm	3 gm	2 mg

Not-Too-Cheesy Cauliflower Soup

Move over green leafy vegetables! This soup is a good source for both vitamins A and C. One serving provides 60% of the US RDA for vitamin A and 85% of the US RDA for vitamin C. After a strenuous workout, try it to replace depleted potassium. One serving gives you 31 times as much potassium as one cup of Gatorade.

> 1-1/2 cups coarsely chopped cauliflower (about
>   1/2 medium-size head)
> 2 small potatoes, peeled, diced (8 oz. *total*)
> 1 medium-size carrot, sliced (4 oz.)
> 1 (14-1/2-oz.) can regular-strength chicken broth *or*
>   1-3/4 cups homemade chicken broth
> 1/2 cup water
> 1/8 teaspoon *each* dry mustard and ground nutmeg
> 1 cup buttermilk
> 2 tablespoons dry sherry
> 3/4 cup shredded sharp Cheddar cheese (3 oz.)
> 1 green onion, thinly sliced, including top

In a 2-quart saucepan, combine cauliflower, potatoes, carrot, chicken broth and water. Bring to a boil over high heat; reduce heat. Cover; simmer 30 minutes or until vegetables are tender. In a blender or food processor, process soup, a portion at a time, until very smooth. Return to pan. Whisk in mustard, nutmeg, buttermilk and sherry. Heat to simmering. Add cheese; stir, and heat just until cheese melts. *Do not allow soup to boil.* Serve in mugs or individual bowls. Garnish with green onion slices. Makes 5 (1-cup) servings.

PER SERVING: 1 cup				
CALORIES	CARBOHYDRATES	PROTEIN	FAT	CHOLESTEROL
170	18 gm	10 gm	7 gm	19 mg

Creamy Chicken-Corn Soup

A creamy stick-to-the-ribs soup without the cream—a real savings on fat and calories. The same amount of homemade corn chowder has twice the calories, three times the fat, and half as much protein. This is a great way for lactose-intolerant people to enjoy a thick, satisfying soup.

> 1/4 teaspoon cornstarch
> 1/4 teaspoon salt
> 1/2 teaspoon dry sherry
> 1 tablespoon water
> 1/2 whole chicken breast, skinned, boned, finely diced (4 oz.)
> 1-1/2 teaspoons vegetable oil
> 1 (17-oz.) can cream-style corn
> 2-1/2 cups homemade chicken broth *or* 1 (14-1/2-oz.) can
>   regular-strength chicken broth plus 3/4 cup water
> 1-1/2 tablespoons cornstarch mixed with 3 tablespoons water
> 1 egg
> 1 green onion, thinly sliced, including top

In a small bowl, combine the 1/4 teaspoon cornstarch, salt, sherry and water. Stir in chicken. Add oil and stir to coat. Let stand, uncovered, 10 minutes. In a 2-quart saucepan, combine corn and chicken broth. Heat to simmering. Stir in chicken. Simmer, uncovered, 5 minutes or until chicken is opaque. Stir cornstarch-water mixture; add to soup. Cook, stirring, until soup comes to a gentle boil and thickens slightly. Remove pan from heat. In a bowl lightly beat egg; while constantly stirring soup, pour in egg. Stir until it forms long threads. Serve soup in individual bowls. Garnish each serving with green onion. Makes 5 (1-cup) servings.

PER SERVING: 1 cup				
CALORIES	CARBOHYDRATES	PROTEIN	FAT	CHOLESTEROL
171	22 gm	12 gm	5 gm	74 mg

Portuguese Sopa

Add a little spice to your life with this hearty whole-meal soup. It provides almost half the US RDA for protein, yet a 1-1/2-cup serving contains less fat than a pat of butter.

> 2 medium-size onions, chopped (10 oz. *total*)
> 4 garlic cloves, pressed *or* minced
> 1 cup dry white wine
> 1 (8-oz.) can tomato sauce
> 2 bay leaves
> 1/2 teaspoon pepper
> 1/2 teaspoon ground cinnamon
> 1/4 teaspoon ground cloves
> 1/4 teaspoon ground cumin
> 1 lb. center-cut beef shank
> 4 cups water
> Salt to taste
> 1 small cabbage (1-1/2 lbs.)
> 3 tablespoons coarsely chopped fresh mint *or*
>   1 tablespoon dried mint

In a 5-quart kettle, combine onions, garlic, wine, tomato sauce, bay leaves, pepper, cinnamon, cloves, cumin and beef shank. Bring to a boil over high heat; reduce heat. Cover; simmer 30 minutes, turning meat several times during cooking. Add water. Continue to simmer 40 minutes or until meat is fork-tender. With a slotted spoon, remove meat to a plate; let cool 5 minutes. Cut meat into bite-size pieces, discarding bone and gristle. Return meat to kettle. Add salt to taste. Cut uncored cabbage in 6 wedges. Press cabbage down into broth. Heat to simmering; cover and simmer 12 minutes or until cabbage is tender. Discard bay leaves. Serve in wide soup bowls. Garnish each serving with mint. Makes 6 (1-1/2-cup) servings.

PER SERVING: 1-1/2 cups

CALORIES	CARBOHYDRATES	PROTEIN	FAT	CHOLESTEROL
269	16 gm	27 gm	8 gm	73 mg

Homemade Chicken Broth

This easy-to-make stock is low in calories, carbohydrates, protein, fat, cholesterol and sodium, yet, it is very high in flavor, and is the best choice for soup making when you want to limit your fat and sodium intake.

> 3 pounds chicken bones (backs, wings)
> 1 large onion, quartered (7 oz.)
> 1 large carrot, cut in chunks (6 oz.)
> 1 large celery stalk, with leaves, sliced
> 4 parsley sprigs
> 1 bay leaf
> 4 whole black peppercorns
> 1/4 teaspoon dried thyme
> 2 whole cloves
> 8 cups cold water

In a large kettle, combine chicken bones, onion, carrot, celery, parsley, bay leaf, peppercorns, thyme, cloves and water. Bring to a boil over high heat; reduce heat. Cover with lid ajar; simmer gently for 2 hours. Strain; discard bones and vegetables. Cool broth; refrigerate until broth is chilled and fat solidifies on surface. Scrape off and discard fat. Use within three days or freeze in 1 cup portions. Makes 4 cups.

PER SERVING: 1 cup				
CALORIES	CARBOHYDRATES	PROTEIN	FAT	CHOLESTEROL
22	2 gm	3 gm	0.5 gm	1 mg

BEEF, PORK, LAMB & VEAL

Meat is one of the main sources for protein, and protein is an important building block for the body. It supplies essential nutrients that keep your complex system in good repair. The catch is that when you eat more protein than your body requires, the surplus becomes an expensive source of calories which are stored as body fat. The American Heart Association recommends that a heart-healthy diet include only two 3-ounce servings of good quality protein a day.

Red meat is becoming leaner. This is good news for the health-conscious eater. While red meat is packed with protein, B vitamins and iron, it contains saturated fat which is especially bad for hearts. A physically active person is not immune to the health risks associated with a high-fat diet. Even a well-conditioned athlete should limit the quantity and type of fat he or she eats. Most of the recipes in this chapter supply no more than 15 grams of fat per serving.

Ranchers are producing leaner breeds, and butchers are trimming more fat from meat before they package it for sale. The USDA recently introduced the term "Lite" for use in the labeling of meat. "Lite" meat is defined as having at least 25% less fat than regular meat. If you cannot find the leaner breeds of beef, or meat labeled as "Lite" in your market, choose cuts that naturally contain less fat. Leaner cuts of meat include: round steak, round roast, sirloin, flank steak, pork loin chops, lamb leg, lamb loin chops, veal steaks, ground veal, veal cutlets and veal chops.

To test meat for doneness, when cooking small pieces of beef, such as in a stir-fry, cook until meat is browned on the outside and still pink within when slashed. If cooking a large piece of beef slash in thickest part; cook rare or until done to your liking. When cooking pork, cook until meat turns white throughout (do not serve pork pink). When cooking lamb, cook until done to your liking.

Albondigas in Chili-Tomato Sauce

South-of-the-border meatballs are known as "albondigas." Making meatballs can be laborious, because they are messy to fry and usually stick to the skillet. Poaching them in a chili-spiked sauce is the traditional no-fuss cooking technique of Mexican cooks. For heart-warming fare, ladle the meatballs and sauce over rice. This is a recipe when the leanest grade of ground beef is the best choice.

1 (8-oz.) can tomatoes
1 cup water
1 to 2 tablespoons chili powder
1/2 teaspoon dried oregano
1/4 teaspoon salt
2 teaspoons vegetable oil
1/4 cup chopped onion
1 small garlic clove, pressed *or* minced
Albondigas (recipe below)
3 cups hot cooked long-grain rice (1 cup uncooked)
1/4 cup low-fat sour cream
2 green onions, thinly sliced, including tops
2 tablespoons chopped cilantro leaves

Albondigas (meatballs):
3/4 lb. extra-lean ground beef
1 egg, lightly beaten
2 tablespoons all-purpose flour
2 tablespoons finely chopped onion
1 small garlic clove, pressed *or* minced
1/4 teaspoon ground cumin
1/4 teaspoon salt

In a blender, combine tomatoes and their liquid, water, chili powder, oregano and salt; process to make a puree and reserve. In a 3-quart saucepan heat oil over medium heat. Add onion and garlic; cook until onion is soft but not browned. Add reserved tomato puree. Heat to simmering; simmer, uncovered, for 15 minutes. Prepare Albondigas. Drop meatballs into simmering sauce; once all are added stir gently to coat. Cook, uncovered, for 5 minutes. Cover pan; simmer 15 minutes or until meatballs are no longer pink in center when slashed and sauce has thickened slightly. Evenly divide rice among 4 wide bowls. Evenly divide meatballs and sauce over rice. Garnish each serving with sour cream, green onions and cilantro. Makes 4 servings.

Albondigas:
In a medium-size bowl, combine meat, egg, flour, onion, garlic, cumin and salt. Mix well. Shape into 16 (1-1/2-inch) balls.

PER SERVING: 1/4 of total recipe				
CALORIES	CARBOHYDRATES	PROTEIN	FAT	CHOLESTEROL
391	47 gm	24 gm	11 gm	121 mg

Caraway-Beef Cabbage Rolls

This is one time when it pays to buy extra-lean ground beef because as the meat cooks inside the cabbage leaves it renders out little fat. Though low in calories, this entree is nutrient-dense, notably with vitamin C, protein and iron. For a Polish feast, accompany this hearty entree with a good dark rye bread and Pickled Beets, page 143, then splurge with a slice of warm Apple Strudel, page 183.

> 1 lb. extra-lean ground beef
> 1 cup uncooked long-grain white rice
> 1/4 cup finely chopped onion
> 1 teaspoon caraway seeds
> 1/2 teaspoon pepper
> 1 (8-oz.) can tomato sauce
> 2 large heads cabbage, cored (about 2-1/2 lbs. *each*)
> 2 (12-oz. *each*) cans vegetable juice cocktail
> 1-1/2 cups plain low-fat yogurt

In a bowl, combine beef, rice, onion, caraway seeds, pepper and tomato sauce. Mix well; set aside. Hold each cabbage head, cored-side-up, under cold running water and gently peel off large leaves one at a time. You will need 28 large leaves. Save small inner hearts of cabbage for salad, if desired. Drop leaves into a large kettle of simmering water; cook for 4 minutes or until leaves are bright green and limp. Lift blanched leaves out with tongs; drain well. Remove V-shaped, thick, white rib at stem end of each leaf to make them easier to roll. To stuff each leaf, mound 2 tablespoons filling at stem and fold in lower edges over filling, then fold in both sides; roll to enclose. Place cabbage rolls, side-by-side, seam-side-down, in two or three layers in a 5-quart kettle. Pour vegetable juice over stuffed rolls. If necessary, add enough water just so cabbage rolls are barely covered with liquid. Place a plate on cabbage rolls to weight them down. Bring to a boil over high heat; reduce heat. Cover; simmer 1 hour. Lift out hot cabbage rolls with a slotted spoon; place on individual plates. Spoon a little of the pan juice over rolls. Top each serving with about 3 tablespoons yogurt. Makes 7 servings of 4 rolls each.

PER SERVING: 4 rolls				
CALORIES	CARBOHYDRATES	PROTEIN	FAT	CHOLESTEROL
294	37 gm	20 gm	6 gm	44 mg

Asparagus-Beef with Black Bean Sauce

For stir-frying, lean flank steak is a good choice. It has little marbling (internal fat) and cooks up tender and juicy. Since flank steak comes in a size larger than you need for one meal (usually two pounds), cut it in half or thirds and freeze. Don't let it thaw completely before slicing. It's easier to cut thin strips of meat that are still frosty and firm. Look for fermented black beans in the Oriental section of the supermarket.

Cooking Sauce (recipe below)
1/2 lb. flank steak
1 teaspoon soy sauce
1-1/2 teaspoons dry sherry
2 teaspoons water
1 teaspoon cornstarch
Dash black pepper
3/4 lb. asparagus
2 tablespoons vegetable oil
1 large garlic clove, pressed *or* minced
1/2 teaspoon minced fresh gingerroot
2 teaspoons fermented black beans, rinsed, drained, finely chopped
1 small onion, cut in wedges, layers separated (3 oz.)
4 large mushrooms, sliced
2 tablespoons water

Cooking Sauce:
1/2 cup water
1 tablespoon cornstarch
1 teaspoon soy sauce

Prepare Cooking Sauce; set aside. Trim any visible fat from meat. Cut meat with the grain in 1-1/2-inch-wide strips, then cut across the grain in 1/8-inch-thick slanting slices. In a medium-size bowl, combine soy sauce, sherry, the 2 teaspoons water, cornstarch and pepper. Add meat; mix well. Let stand, uncovered, for 15 minutes. Snap off tough asparagus ends; cut in 1-1/2-inch slanting slices. Heat a wok or large skillet over high heat. When pan is hot, add 1 tablespoon of the oil. When oil is hot, add garlic, gingerroot, and black beans; stir once. Add beef; stir-fry for 1-1/2 minutes or until meat is browned on the outside but still pink within. Remove meat from pan. Heat the remaining 1 tablespoon oil. Add asparagus, onion and mushrooms. Stir-fry for 30 seconds. Add the 2 tablespoons water; cover pan. Cook for 2 minutes or until vegetables are crisp-tender. Return meat to pan. Stir through cooking sauce once to recombine; add to pan. Cook, stirring, until sauce bubbles and thickens. Makes 3 servings.

Cooking Sauce:
In a small bowl, combine water, cornstarch and soy sauce; stir until cornstarch dissolves.

PER SERVING: 1/3 of total recipe

CALORIES	CARBOHYDRATES	PROTEIN	FAT	CHOLESTEROL
278	9 gm	26 gm	15 gm	71 mg

Bahmie Goreng

Bahmie Goreng (Indonesian fried noodles) is a delicious example of the Asian knack of stretching a small amount of protein with a starch. One serving supplies half the amount of protein you need each day. Cabbage provides vitamin C and contains components which are thought to inhibit the development of cancer.

2 tablespoons instant minced onion
8 oz. fettucini, broken in half
1/2 lb. flank steak
2 tablespoons vegetable oil
2 garlic cloves, pressed *or* minced
1/2 teaspoon crushed red pepper
1/4 lb. medium-size raw shrimp, shelled, deveined
1 medium-size onion, cut in half lengthwise, thinly sliced
**   crosswise (5 oz.)**
2 celery stalks, thinly sliced (1 cup)
1/2 small red bell pepper, seeded, cored, cut in
**   3/4-inch squares (half 4 oz.)**
1/3 cup regular-strength chicken broth
2 cups coarsely chopped cabbage (1/2 small head)
1 tablespoon soy sauce

In a small dry skillet, place instant minced onion. Place over medium heat; cook 30 to 60 seconds or until onion is toasted. Remove pan from heat; set aside and let cool. In a large kettle of boiling water, cook fettucini 8 to 10 minutes or until tender but firm to the bite; drain. Rinse with cold water, drain again; set aside. Meanwhile, trim any visible fat from meat. Cut across the grain in 1/8-inch-thick slanting slices; set aside. Heat a wok or large skillet over high heat. When pan is hot, add 1 tablespoon of the oil. When oil is hot, add garlic and red pepper; stir once. Add beef strips; stir-fry for 1 minute. Add shrimp; stir-fry just until shrimp turn pink and meat is browned on the outside but still pink within. Remove meat and shrimp from pan. Heat the remaining 1 tablespoon oil. Add onion, celery and bell pepper. Stir-fry for 30 seconds. Add 2 tablespoons of the broth; cover pan. Cook for 2 minutes or until vegetables are crisp-tender. Add cabbage and 2 more tablespoons of the broth; stir-fry for 2 minutes. Add cooked fettucini, the remaining broth and soy sauce. Stir-fry for 1 minute. Return meat and shrimp to pan. Stir-fry until most of liquid has evaporated. Evenly divide among 4 plates. Sprinkle toasted minced onion over each serving. Makes 4 servings.

PER SERVING: 1/4 of total recipe

CALORIES	CARBOHYDRATES	PROTEIN	FAT	CHOLESTEROL
393	42 gm	29 gm	12 gm	94 mg

Singapore Saté

In Southeast Asia, a favorite street fare meal is bites of marinated meat threaded on bamboo skewers, then cooked on a grill. It's called saté (sahtay) and it makes a wonderful partner to rice. Plan on four ounces of meat per serving and use any of the suggestions for meat that you like. If you use bamboo skewers, to prevent them from burning on the grill, soak them for 30 minutes in water before threading meat. Serve with Grilled Eggplant, page 145.

> 2 tablespoon soy sauce
> 2 tablespoons lime juice
> 1 tablespoon packed brown sugar
> 2 garlic cloves, minced *or* pressed
> 1/2 teaspoon ground coriander
> 1/4 teaspoon ground cumin
> 1/2 teaspoon grated fresh gingerroot
> 1/4 teaspoon pepper
> 1-1/2 lbs. lean boneless beef (such as London broil) *or*
>   leg of lamb *or* pork loin

In a bowl, combine soy sauce, lime juice, brown sugar, garlic, coriander, cumin, ginger and pepper; stir until sugar dissolves. Cut meat in 3/4-inch cubes; place in a plastic bag. Pour marinade over meat; seal bag. Turn bag to distribute marinade; refrigerator for 2 hours. Remove meat from marinade; reserve marinade. Thread about 4 cubes of meat on each of about 18 small skewers. Preheat grill. Grease grill with vegetable nonstick cooking spray. Place skewers on grill 4 to 6 inches above a solid bed of medium-glowing coals. Cook, turning often, for 8 to 10 minutes; brush occasionally with marinade during cooking. Cook beef or lamb until meat is browned on the outside and still pink within when slashed and pork is white throughout (pork should not be pink when cut). Makes 6 servings.

PER SERVING: 1/6 of total recipe				
CALORIES	CARBOHYDRATES	PROTEIN	FAT	CHOLESTEROL
239	3 gm	31 gm	16 gm	99 mg

Mexican Stir-Fry

Stir-frying is a marvelously fast technique when you cook for a few. That doesn't mean you must limit yourself to using Chinese seasonings every time you pull out the wok. This entree is spirited with Mexican flavors, the perfect accompaniment to a bowl of steamed rice. You can cut up the remaining jicama to add crunch to a salad another day.

1 tablespoon lime juice
1/2 teaspoon ground cumin
1/2 teaspoon dried oregano
1/2 teaspoon salt
1/2 lb. flank steak
2 teaspoons cornstarch
1/2 cup regular-strength chicken broth
5 teaspoons vegetable oil
2 large garlic cloves, pressed *or* minced
2 teaspoons fermented black beans, rinsed, drained,
   finely chopped
2 small fresh Serrano *or* jalapeno chiles, seeded, finely
   chopped, *or* 1/2 teaspoon crushed red pepper
1 medium-size onion, cut in wedges, layers separated (5 oz.)
1/2 small jicama, cut in 1/4-inch julienne strips (1 cup)
1 medium-size red bell pepper, seeded, cored,
   cut in 1/4-inch-wide strips (6 oz.)
2 small zucchini, cut in 1/4-inch-thick slanting
   slices (8 oz. *total*)
1/2 (15-oz.) can whole baby sweet corn, drained,
   cut in half lengthwise

In a medium-size bowl, combine lime juice, cumin, oregano and salt. Trim any visible fat from meat. Cut across the grain in 1/8-inch-thick slanting slices. Add meat slices; mix well. Let stand, uncovered, for 15 minutes. In a small bowl, combine cornstarch and 1/4 cup of the chicken broth; set aside. Heat a wok or large skillet over high heat. When pan is hot, add 3 teaspoons of the oil. When oil is hot, add garlic, black beans and chiles; stir once. Add meat; stir-fry for 1-1/2 minutes or until meat is browned on the outside but still pink within. Remove meat from pan. Heat the remaining 2 teaspoons oil. Add onion and jicama. Stir-fry for 30 seconds. Add 2 tablespoons of the chicken broth; cover pan. Cook for 2 minutes. Add bell pepper, zucchini and the remaining 2 tablespoons chicken broth. Cover; cook for 2 minutes or until vegetables are crisp-tender. Return meat to pan. Add baby corn. Stir through cornstarch-chicken broth mixture once to recombine; add to pan. Cook stirring, until sauce bubbles and thickens slightly. Makes 3 servings.

PER SERVING: 1/3 of total recipe				
CALORIES	CARBOHYDRATES	PROTEIN	FAT	CHOLESTEROL
361	33 gm	28 gm	13 gm	71 mg

Burrito Grande

Diced eggplant and potato mingle with beef in this unusual Mexican entree. Add a crisp green salad and you have a complete meal.

Burrito Grande Filling (recipe below)
1 dozen (8-inch) whole-wheat flour tortillas *or*
   regular flour tortillas
1 cup shredded farmer cheese (4 oz.)
1/2 cup low-fat sour cream
3 green onions, thinly sliced, including tops

Burrito Grande Filling:
1/2 teaspoon salt
1/2 lb. lean ground beef
1 small onion, chopped (3 oz.)
1 garlic clove, pressed *or* minced
1/2 eggplant, peeled, cut in 1/2-inch dice (half 1 lb.)
2 medium-size potatoes, peeled, cut in dice (12 oz. *total*)
1/2 cup tomato sauce
1/2 cup water
1 teaspoon chili powder
1/4 teaspoon ground cumin
1/8 teaspoon pepper

Prepare Burrito Grand Filling; keep warm. Preheat oven to 350F (175C). Remove paper separators between tortillas, if necessary; stack and wrap tortillas in foil. Heat in oven 15 minutes. Grease a shallow 15″ x 10″ rimmed baking pan with vegetable nonstick cooking spray; set aside. Remove tortillas from oven. Place 1/3 cup hot filling in center of each tortilla. Roll up. Place burritos, seam-side-down, in prepared pan. Sprinkle cheese evenly over burritos. Broil 6 inches from heat until cheese melts. Place 2 burritos on each of six plates. Garnish each burrito with 2 teaspoons of sour cream and a sprinkle of green onion. Makes 6 servings, 2 burritos each.

Burrito Grande Filling:
Sprinkle salt in a large skillet with a lid. Place over medium-high heat. Crumble in beef; cook until browned. Add onion and garlic. Reduce heat to medium; cook until onion is soft but not browned. Discard drippings. Add eggplant, potatoes, tomato sauce, water, chili powder, cumin and pepper. Heat to simmering. Cover; simmer 25 to 30 minutes, stirring twice during cooking, or until potatoes are fork-tender. Makes 4 cups.

PER SERVING: 2 burritos

CALORIES	CARBOHYDRATES	PROTEIN	FAT	CHOLESTEROL
362	50 gm	18 gm	10 gm	38 mg

Fajitas

Wrap strips of grilled beef and Mexican garnishes inside a tortilla for a tasty entree that has a high ratio of vitamins and minerals in relation to calories. One serving supplies 67% of the protein, 32% of the niacin, and 27% of the iron you need each day. Serve a shredded lettuce, tomato and radish salad on the side. Flank steak should be served rare or medium-rare. If cooked to the well done stage, the meat becomes tough.

>1 (1-1/4 lbs.) flank steak
>1/4 cup lime juice
>2 tablespoons tequila
>2 garlic cloves, pressed *or* minced
>1/2 teaspoon salt
>1/4 teaspoon pepper
>6 (8-inch) flour tortillas
>1/2 cup Guacamole, page 53
>1/2 cup low-fat sour cream
>1/2 cup Roasted Sweet Pepper Salsa, page 55

Trim any visible fat from meat. Place meat in a plastic bag. Add lime juice, tequila, garlic, salt and pepper; seal bag. Turn bag to distribute marinade. Marinate in refrigerator for 8 hours or as long as overnight; turn bag once to distribute marinade. Preheat grill. Remove paper separators between tortillas if necessary; stack and wrap tortillas in foil. Grease grill with vegetable nonstick cooking spray. Place tortillas on side of grill to heat. Remove meat from marinade. Place meat on grill 4 to 6 inches above a solid bed of medium-glowing coals. Grill 4 minutes on each side for rare or until meat is brown on the outside but still pink within; meat should still be pink when slashed in thickest part. To serve, cut meat across the grain in thin slanting slices. Unwrap tortillas, place a few meat slices down center of each tortilla. Top with guacamole, sour cream and salsa. Fold up to enclose. Makes 6 servings.

PER SERVING: 1/6 of total recipe

CALORIES	CARBOHYDRATES	PROTEIN	FAT	CHOLESTEROL
333	23 gm	31 gm	13 gm	89 mg

Quick Moussaka

You can make the filling one day ahead. Take a jog, bike ride or work out in the gym, then just assemble and pop this creamy custard casserole in the oven and relax while it bakes. Serve with hot noodles.

>1 recipe Burrito Grande Filling, page 81
>2 eggs
>1 cup plain low-fat yogurt (8 oz.)

Grease a 1-quart casserole with vegetable nonstick cooking spray; set aside. Prepare Burrito Grande Filling; place in prepared casserole. Cool, cover and refrigerate, if made ahead. To bake, preheat oven to 350F (175C). In a bowl, beat eggs slightly. Add yogurt; whisk until evenly blended. Pour over meat mixture; spread out to edge of dish. Bake, uncovered, in preheated oven 45 minutes (55 minutes if refrigerated) or until a knife inserted in center of topping comes out clean. Remove from oven. Let stand 5 minutes before serving. Makes 4 servings.

PER SERVING: 1/4 of total recipe

CALORIES	CARBOHYDRATES	PROTEIN	FAT	CHOLESTEROL
264	26 gm	21 gm	8 gm	162 mg

New Joe's Special

Popeye would be proud of this dish. Not only is it loaded with iron-rich chard (or spinach), it contains red meat and tofu, both extremely high in iron. As a bonus, the beef in this recipe increases the absorption of the iron from the greens. Serve it with steamed brown or white rice and broiled tomato halves. It is not necessary to use extra-lean ground beef in this recipe because the fatty pan drippings can be easily discarded after the ground beef has browned.

> 5 large red *or* green Swiss chard stalks (1/2 lb.) *or*
>   1 bunch spinach (12 oz.)
> 1/4 teaspoon salt
> 2/3 lb. lean ground beef
> 1 medium-size onion, chopped (5 oz.)
> 1 garlic clove, pressed *or* minced
> 1/4 teaspoon dried oregano
> 1/8 teaspoon pepper
> 1 tablespoon soy sauce
> 1/3 pkg. regular *or* firm tofu, rinsed, patted dry (14 to 16 oz.)

Wash and drain chard stalks. Cut off heavy chard stems; finely chop and place in a bowl; set aside. Coarsely chop chard leaves, place in another bowl and set aside. (If using spinach, remove and discard stems; wash, drain, coarsely chop leaves and set aside.) Sprinkle salt in a 5-quart kettle over medium-high heat. Crumble in beef; cook until browned, then discard drippings. Add onion, garlic and chopped chard stems. Reduce heat to medium. Cook 8 minutes; stir occasionally or until onion is soft but not browned. Add chard leaves, oregano, pepper and soy sauce; stir until well mixed. Finely crumble tofu into kettle. Heat to simmering; cover. Simmer 5 minutes or until chard leaves are wilted. Makes 4 (1-cup) servings.

PER SERVING: 1 cup

CALORIES	CARBOHYDRATES	PROTEIN	FAT	CHOLESTEROL
187	7 gm	20 gm	9 gm	49 mg

Hurry-Up Chili With Beans

Whip up a bowl-of-red that's packed with fire, flavor and fiber. It's an excellent source for protein, iron and the B-vitamins. One serving supplies 69% of the US RDA for vitamin C and 28% of the US RDA for iron. You can get rid of the saturated-fat drippings with a bulb baster, but draining the meat in a colander does a more thorough job.

1-1/2 lbs. lean ground beef
1 tablespoon vegetable oil
2 large onions, chopped (1 lb. *total*)
4 garlic cloves, pressed *or* minced
1 medium-size green bell pepper, seeded, cored,
  chopped (6 oz.)
2 tablespoons chili powder
2 teaspoons ground cumin
1 teaspoon dried oregano
1/4 to 1/2 teaspoon red (cayenne) pepper
1/4 teaspoon ground cinnamon
2 (16-oz. *each*) cans whole peeled tomatoes
1/4 cup tomato paste
1 (12-oz.) can beer
6 cups cooked pinto beans *or* kidney beans *or*
  2 (27-oz. *each*) cans kidney beans, drained
Salt and pepper to taste

Garnishes:
4 green onions, thinly sliced, including tops
3/4 cup shredded Cheddar cheese (3 oz.)
1/2 cup plain low-fat yogurt *or* low-fat sour cream
2 limes *or* lemons, cut in wedges
1/2 cup Ten-Minute Salsa, page 56, *or* commercially
  prepared salsa

Heat a 5-quart kettle over medium-high heat. Crumble in beef; cook until browned. Remove kettle from heat. Set a colander over a large bowl. Pour meat into colander; let fat drain. Meanwhile, return kettle to medium heat; add oil. When oil is hot, add onions, garlic and bell pepper; cook until onion is soft but not browned. Stir in chili powder, cumin, oregano, red pepper and cinnamon; cook 1 minute. Pour tomatoes and their liquid into kettle; coarsely cut up tomatoes. Stir in tomato paste until well blended. Add drained meat, beer and beans; mix well. Heat to simmering. Cover; simmer 30 minutes or until flavors blend. Add salt and pepper to taste. Place garnishes in individual bowls; pass at the table to spoon over each serving. Makes 8 (1-1/2-cup) servings.

PER SERVING: 1-1/2 cups				
CALORIES	CARBOHYDRATES	PROTEIN	FAT	CHOLESTEROL
447	49 gm	34 gm	15 gm	69 mg

Green Chile Stew

You don't need to be a top-seeded sprinter to want energy, and here is a way to enhance it. This stew is chock-full of protein, thiamin, and iron plus a high amount of vitamin C which increases the absorption of the iron. Serve it over pinto beans, hominy, rice or baked potato as the filler-upper.

   2 lbs. lean boneless pork butt
   2-1/2 cups water
   1 large onion, chopped (7 oz.)
   2 garlic cloves, pressed *or* minced
   1 (16-oz.) can whole peeled tomatoes
   2 tablespoons tomato paste
   2 (7-oz. *each*) cans whole green chiles, cut in 1-inch squares
   1/4 teaspoon ground cumin
   Salt and pepper to taste

Trim any visible fat from meat, then cut in 1-inch cubes. Place pork and 1/2 cup of the water in a 5-quart kettle; cover. Bring to a boil over high heat. Reduce heat; cover and simmer 20 minutes. Uncover, increase heat to high; cook until liquid evaporates. When meat starts to sizzle in its own fat, stir frequently until it is lightly browned. Reduce heat to medium. Add onion and garlic. Cook until onion is soft but not browned. Add tomatoes and their liquid; coarsely cut up tomatoes. Stir to loosen any browned bits from kettle bottom. Stir in tomato paste until well blended. Add chiles, cumin and the remaining 2 cups water. Bring to a boil over high heat. Reduce heat. Cover; simmer 1 hour or until meat is fork-tender. Uncover; simmer 10 minutes or until sauce thickens slightly. Add salt and pepper to taste. Makes 8 (1-cup) servings.

PER SERVING: 1 cup				
CALORIES	CARBOHYDRATES	PROTEIN	FAT	CHOLESTEROL
295	10 gm	30 gm	15 gm	95 mg

Pork Ragout

This savory, robust stew contributes many nutrients, but is especially high in protein, the primary structural material for your body, vitamin C and iron. One serving supplies 1/4 of the amount of iron that a woman needs each day. It tastes great after a day on the slopes. Serve it over noodles to soak up the savory juices.

1-1/2 lbs. lean boneless pork butt
1/2 cup water
1 tablespoon vegetable oil
2 medium-size onions, cut in half lengthwise, thinly sliced
 crosswise (5 oz. *each*)
1 (16-oz.) can whole peeled tomatoes
1 medium-size green bell pepper, seeded, cored, cut into
 thin strips (6 oz.)
2 teaspoons paprika
1/2 teaspoon dried thyme
1/2 teaspoon dried marjoram
1 bay leaf
1 teaspoon caraway seeds
Red (cayenne) pepper to taste
1 cup regular-strength beef broth
1 (16-oz.) can sauerkraut
1/2 cup plain low-fat yogurt

Trim pork butt of all visible fat. Cut in 1-inch cubes. Place pork and water in a 5-quart kettle; cover. Bring to a boil over high heat. Reduce heat; cover and simmer for 20 minutes. Uncover; increase heat to high. Cook, stirring occasionally, until liquid evaporates. Continue to cook until meat is browned. Remove meat from kettle. Add oil. Place over medium heat. When oil is hot, add onions; cook until onions are soft but not browned. Stir to loosen any browned bits from kettle bottom. Pour tomatoes and their liquid into kettle; coarsely cut up tomatoes. Return meat to kettle. Add bell pepper, paprika, thyme, marjoram, bay leaf, caraway seeds, red pepper to taste and broth; stir to combine ingredients. Bring to a boil over high heat; reduce heat. Cover; simmer 1 hour or until meat is fork-tender. Pour sauerkraut into a colander; rinse well under running tap water. With cupped hands, squeeze sauerkraut dry. Add to kettle; stir lightly to mix. Cover and cook for 5 minutes or until heated through. Discard bay leaf. Place yogurt in a serving dish; pass at the table to spoon over each serving. Makes 7 (1-cup) servings.

PER SERVING: 1/7 of total recipe				
CALORIES	CARBOHYDRATES	PROTEIN	FAT	CHOLESTEROL
312	11 gm	30 gm	16 gm	89 mg

Tofu-Pork in Oyster Sauce

Japanese cooks are masters at combining slivers of meat with tofu. It's an easy way to stretch flavor and double the protein without doubling the fat. Serve this iron-rich entree over rice cooked in the Oriental style, without salt and without fat, and pass a bowl of sliced cucumbers dressed with purchased, seasoned rice vinegar for a cool accent.

> 1 (14- to 16-oz.) pkg. regular *or* firm tofu, rinsed, patted dry
> 3/4 cup water
> 2 tablespoons dry sherry
> 2 teaspoons soy sauce
> Dash red (cayenne) pepper
> 2 teaspoon vegetable oil
> 1/2 lb. lean boneless pork, cut in strips 1/4-inch thick,
>   1/2-inch wide, 1-1/2 inches long
> 1/2 teaspoon grated fresh gingerroot
> 1 large onion, cut in half lengthwise, sliced crosswise in
>   1/4-inch-thick slices (7 oz.)
> 1/4 lb. Chinese pea pods, ends and side strings removed
> 5 green onions, cut in 1-1/2-inch diagonal slices,
>   including tops
> 2 teaspoons cornstarch mixed with 1 tablespoon water
> 2 tablespoons oyster sauce

Cut tofu in domino-shape pieces 1-1/2 inches long, 3/4-inch wide and 1/4-inch thick; place in a colander to drain. In a small bowl, combine water, sherry, soy sauce and red pepper; set aside. In a large skillet with a nonstick finish, heat oil over medium heat. Add pork and ginger. Cook meat for 2 minutes on each side or until meat turns white throughout. Add onion slices; cook 2 minutes. Push meat to one side of skillet; add tofu. Spoon meat over tofu; gently combine. Pour water-sherry mixture over meat. Reduce heat to low. Simmer, uncovered, 5 minutes. Add Chinese peas and green onions; cover. Simmer 2 minutes. Stir through cornstarch and water once to recombine; add to skillet. Cook, stirring around edge to avoid breaking up tofu, until sauce bubbles and thickens slightly. Stir in oyster sauce; heat through. Makes 4 servings.

PER SERVING: 1/4 of total recipe

CALORIES	CARBOHYDRATES	PROTEIN	FAT	CHOLESTEROL
278	13 gm	25 gm	15 gm	50 mg

Purchasing & Storing Fresh Gingerroot:
Purchase fresh gingerroot in small qualtities; if you can only find large pieces, break off a small knob. To store, wrap gingerroot in a dry paper towel and enclose in a plastic bag; store in refrigerator for up to 2 weeks. Or for longer storage, peel gingerroort and cut in 1/8-inch-thick slices. Place in a small jar with a lid. Cover with dry sherry; refrigerate up to 6 months. The sherry picks up the ginger flavor and is a nice addition to a stir-fry dish.

Mushroom-Veal Loaf

One serving of this mushroom-studded loaf supplies over 100% of the amount of niacin you need each day. Plus, it's a good source of iron and B vitamins which work together to break down carbohydrates and turn them into energy. Serve it hot or cut it in thin 1/4-inch thick slices to serve as a sandwich filling.

2 slices French bread, cut 1/2-inch thick
1/2 cup skim milk
2 tablespoons margarine
1 small onion, chopped (3 oz.)
1 garlic clove, pressed *or* minced
1/4 cup finely diced celery
1/2 lb. small mushrooms, very thinly sliced
2 lbs. ground veal
1 egg
1 teaspoon salt
1/4 teaspoon pepper
1/2 teaspoon dried dill
1/4 teaspoon ground nutmeg

Preheat oven to 400F (205C). Into a large bowl tear bread and crusts into small pieces. In a small pan, heat milk to scalding; pour over bread. Let stand until cool. In a large skillet melt margarine over medium heat. Add onion, garlic and celery; cook until onion is soft but not browned. Add mushrooms. Increase heat to medium-high; cooking until liquid evaporates. Let cool. Squeeze softened bread with your hands to make a smooth pulpy mixture; blend in veal, egg, salt, pepper, dill and nutmeg. Add mushroom mixture; mix well. Spoon into a 9" x 5" loaf pan; spread even. Bake in preheated oven 1 hour or until juices run clear when a knife is inserted in center. Remove pan from oven and cool 5 minutes. Skim off fat. To serve hot, cut loaf in 1/2-inch thick slices. Or cool, cover and refrigerate meatloaf. Cut into 1/4-inch thick slices for a cold meat tray or sandwich filling. Makes 8 servings; 2 slices each 1/2-inch thick *or* 16 servings, 2 slices each 1/4-inch thick.

PER SERVING: 2 (1/2-inch-thick) slices

CALORIES	CARBOHYDRATES	PROTEIN	FAT	CHOLESTEROL
247	8 gm	38 gm	7 gm	144 mg

Storing Fresh Mushrooms:
Store unwashed mushrooms in a paper bag; a plastic bag traps moisture and makes them soft and slippery. Before using, wash mushrooms by quickly dipping them in a bowl of cold water, or place mushrooms in a colander and mist with a fine water spray. There is no need to peel mushrooms; trim stems only if ends are dark.

Veal Patties with Mustard Sauce

Because it comes from very young beef calves, veal has no marbling (internal fat) and very little external fat. For an easy dinner, serve these patties with noodles and Peas with Onions, page 147.

> 1 lb. ground veal
> 1 egg
> 1/4 cup fine dry bread crumbs
> 2 tablespoons skim milk
> 1 garlic clove, pressed *or* minced
> 2 tablespoons chopped parsley
> 1/2 teaspoon salt
> 1/8 teaspoon white pepper
> 1/2 teaspoon dried sage, crumbled
> 1/8 teaspoon ground nutmeg
> 1 tablespoon margarine
> 1/4 cup dry white wine
> 1 tablespoon Dijon-style mustard
> 1/2 cup plain low-fat yogurt

In a large bowl, combine veal, egg, bread crumbs, milk, garlic, parsley, salt, pepper, sage and nutmeg; mix well. Divide mixture into 4 equal portions; lightly shape each portion into a patty 3/4-to 1-inch thick. In a skillet melt margarine over medium-high heat. Place patties in skillet; cook for 5 minutes on each side or until lightly browned and juices run clear when slashed. Remove patties to a serving plate; cover and keep warm. Add wine to skillet; bring to a boil over high heat, scraping up brown bits. Boil until wine is reduced by half; reduce heat to low. Add mustard and yogurt. Whisk until evenly blended and hot; *do not boil.* Spoon sauce over each patty. Makes 4 servings.

PER SERVING: 1 patty				
CALORIES	CARBOHYDRATES	PROTEIN	FAT	CHOLESTEROL
264	8 gm	40 gm	8 gm	156 mg

Lamb Pilaf

For a second performance from a leg of lamb, try this iron-rich pilaf. Serve it with Artichokes Stuffed with Tomato-Eggplant Salad, page 157, or stuff it in pocket bread halves and garnish with chopped tomato, a pickle slice and a spoonful of yogurt.

1 tablespoon vegetable oil
1 medium-size onion, chopped (5 oz.)
2 celery stalks, sliced (1 cup)
1 garlic clove, pressed *or* minced
1/2 teaspoon ground corinader
1/2 teaspoon ground cumin
2 cups diced cooked lamb
4 cups cooked brown *or* white long-grain rice
  (1-1/3 cups uncooked)
1/4 cup chopped parsley
1/4 cup sunflower seeds
1/4 cup regular-strength beef broth *or* regular-strength
  chicken broth
Salt and pepper to taste

In a 5-quart kettle heat oil over medium heat. Add onion, celery and garlic; cook until onion is soft but not browned. Stir in coriander, cumin and lamb; cook for 2 minutes. Add rice, parsley, sunflower seeds and broth. Stir until evenly mixed. Reduce heat to low. Cover; cook for 5 minutes or until rice is heated through and liquid is absorbed. Add salt and pepper to taste. Makes 5 (1-1/3-cup) servings.

PER SERVING: 1-1/3 cups

CALORIES	CARBOHYDRATES	PROTEIN	FAT	CHOLESTEROL
466	42 gm	33 gm	17 gm	74 mg

Grilled Persian Lamb

Unless you just want to add more fuel to smoke up the barbecue, don't add oil to a meat marinade. Meat has enough built-in fat to keep it from drying out when it is grilled. Here is a marvelous marinade for lamb that does all that is required—maximize flavor and tenderness. If you do not find a whole lamb loin ask your butcher to cut you one or use boned leg of lamb.

>   1/2 cup plain low-fat yogurt
>   1/2 cup chopped onion
>   2 garlic cloves, pressed *or* minced
>   1/2 teaspoon salt
>   1/8 teaspoon pepper
>   1/2 teaspoon ground cumin
>   1 tablespoon chopped cilantro leaves
>   2 drops hot pepper sauce
>   1-1/2 lbs. boneless lamb loin *or* leg

In a bowl, combine yogurt, onion, garlic, salt, pepper, cumin, cilantro and hot pepper sauce; mix well. Place lamb in a plastic bag. Pour marinade over lamb; seal bag. Turn bag over to distribute marinade. Marinate in refrigerator for 8 hours or as long as overnight. Preheat grill; lightly grease with vegetable nonstick cooking spray. Pour marinade into a small pan. Place lamb on grill 4 to 6 inches above a solid bed of medium-glowing coals. Grill 5 to 7 minutes on each side for medium-rare or until a meat thermometer reaches 150F (65C) or until done to your liking. Meanwhile, heat marinade on low heat *(do not boil)*. Slice meat into 1/2-inch-thick slices. Pour warm marinade into a serving bowl and pass at the table to spoon over each serving. Makes 6 servings.

PER SERVING: 1/6 of total recipe				
CALORIES	CARBOHYDRATES	PROTEIN	FAT	CHOLESTEROL
226	3 gm	33 gm	8 gm	111 mg

Purchasing & Storing Cilantro:
To store cilantro remove the string around the bunch. Stand cilantro, stem-ends-down, in a glass of water. Cover with a plastic bag and refrigerate up to a week. To use, wash leaves in cold water and pat dry. Discard heavy stems.

Pocket Bread Shish Kebabs

Here's a lean Middle-Eastern style burger with the works. The Lemony Tomato Salad, high in vitamin C, is so refreshing you might want to serve it another time as a side dish with grilled chicken or fish. The kebabs would be equally delicious served with tomato, lettuce and relish. After a good swim, two of these will suffice.

Lemony Tomato Salad (recipe below)
1 lb. lean ground beef *or* ground lamb
1/3 cup finely chopped onion
1/3 cup chopped parsley
1/2 teaspoon salt
1/4 teaspoon ground allspice
About 1/2 cup plain low-fat yogurt
4 (6-inch) regular *or* whole-wheat pocket breads

Lemony Tomato Salad:
1/2 medium-size cucumber, peeled, seeded,
**   coarsely chopped (half 8 oz.)**
2 medium-size tomatoes, coarsely chopped (10 oz. *total*)
1/2 small green bell pepper, seeded, cored,
**   coarsely chopped (half 4 oz.)**
6 radishes, coarsely chopped
2 green onions, thinly sliced, including tops
2 tablespoons chopped parsley
2 teaspoons chopped fresh mint *or* 1 teaspoon
**   dried mint, crumbled**
1 small garlic clove, pressed *or* minced
1 tablespoon olive oil
2 tablespoons lemon juice
Salt and pepper to taste

Prepare Lemony Tomato Salad. In a large bowl, combine beef, onion, parsley, salt, allspice and 2 tablespoons of the yogurt; mix well. Divide meat into 8 equal parts. On work surface, press each part into a patty, 6 inches long and 1-1/2 inches wide. Place a metal skewer lengthwise in center of each patty. Fold sides of patty over skewer; pinch to seal. Gently roll skewer to shape meat into a round cylinder. When all skewers are filled, place in a baking pan. Cover and refrigerate for 30 minutes or as long as 8 hours. Preheat oven to 200F (95C). Cut pocket breads in half crosswise to make 8 half pockets; stack breads and wrap in foil. Place wrapped pocket breads in preheated oven; warm 5 minutes. Remove from oven; set aside. Preheat grill or broiler; lightly grease with vegetable nonstick cooking spray. If grilling, arrange skewers on grill 4 to 6 inches above a solid bed of low-glowing coals. If broiling, arrange skewers 4 inches from heat. Cook meat about 4 minutes or until lightly browned; turn skewers over. Cook 2 to 3 more minutes or until meat is no longer pink when slashed. To serve, open each pocket bread half. Slide shish kebabs off skewers into pocket bread halves. Spoon 1/4 cup Lemony Tomato Salad over each kebab. Top each with about 2 teaspoons yogurt. Makes 8 servings.

Lemony Tomato Salad:
In a large bowl, combine cucumber, tomatoes, bell pepper and radishes; mix well. Add green onions, parsley, mint, garlic, olive oil, lemon juice and salt and pepper to taste; stir well. Cover and refrigerate up to 1 day. Makes 2 cups.

PER SERVING: 1/8 of total recipe

CALORIES	CARBOHYDRATES	PROTEIN	FAT	CHOLESTEROL
207	17 gm	16 gm	9 gm	38 mg

CHICKEN & TURKEY

As a source of high-quality protein, chicken and turkey have a lot in their favor. They are nutrient-dense with a high ratio of vitamins and minerals in relation to calories, low in sodium and low in saturated fats and cholesterol. As if that weren't enough, poultry is economical to buy, easy to cook and adaptable enough to taste good with everything from garlic to grapes.

Not long ago most chickens were only sold whole. Most chicken today is sold in parts so you can tailor your shopping to fit the recipe. While it is more economical to bone poultry yourself, you can buy boned breasts and thighs when time is a factor. Try boned thighs for grilled Tandoori Chicken, page 97, or boned breasts for Chicken Breasts with Hot Marmalade Sauce, page 99, or Stir-Fried Chicken with Vegetables, page 103.

The sale of turkey parts allows you to take advantage of turkey breast, the leanest type of poultry. Boned and sliced into cutlets, it tastes delicious as Turkey Scallopine with Peas, page 107, or Fontina Turkey with Tomato-Basil Sauce, page 106.

Like fish, fresh poultry is perishable and should be cooked within two days after purchasing. If poultry is frozen, let it thaw in its original wrapper in the refrigerator—not at room temperature. To test poultry for doneness, when cooking a whole bird, cook until meat near thigh is no longer pink when slashed. If cooking the breast, the meat should no longer be pink when cut in the thickest part. When you cook bite-size pieces of chicken breast in a stir-fry, the meat should be white rather than opaque.

Roast Chicken with Garlic

After roasting, discard the chicken skin and smear the meat with the sweet-flavored buttery garlic. If you bake potatoes to serve with the chicken, you may want to roast another garlic head to serve as their topper. Compared to the same amount of beef sirloin, 1 serving of this recipe has 300 fewer calories, half the amount of total fat and 10% less saturated fat.

> 1 broiler-fryer chicken (3 lbs.)
> 1/2 teaspoon salt
> 1/2 teaspoon pepper
> 1 celery stalk, cut in half
> 4 parsley sprigs
> 1 bay leaf
> 1 whole garlic head, unpeeled
> 1/4 cup dry white wine
> 1 tablespoon vegetable oil

Remove giblets from chicken and reserve for other uses. Pull off and discard lumps of fat from cavity; rinse chicken and pat dry. Tuck wings under body akimbo-style. Season chicken inside and out with salt and pepper. Place celery, parsley and bay leaf in body cavity. Place chicken, breast-side-up, on a rack in a shallow roasting pan. Place whole garlic head on rack next to chicken. In a small bowl, combine wine and oil; generously brush over chicken only. Roast, uncovered, in a 375F (190C) oven 1 to 1-1/4 hours, or until meat near thigh bone is no longer pink when slashed; baste chicken and garlic several times during the last 30 minutes of cooking. Lift chicken to a warm platter or board to carve. Remove and discard chicken skin, celery, parsley and bay leaf. Cut chicken into serving portions and place on a serving platter. Separate individual cloves of garlic; place in a bowl. Pass garlic at the table. Squeeze garlic from its paper husk onto chicken pieces; spread over meat. Makes 6 servings.

PER SERVING: 1/6 of total recipe				
CALORIES	CARBOHYDRATES	PROTEIN	FAT	CHOLESTEROL
328	1 gm	43 gm	15 gm	132 mg

Crusty Baked Chicken

Coating chicken with seasoned bread crumbs and baking it is a delicious way to duplicate fried chicken without the mess and without the fat. Here are two different coatings to use when time is short. Each recipe can be doubled to serve a crowd.

> **6 *each* chicken legs and thighs (3 lbs. *total*), skin removed**
> **Herbed Blue Cheese Coating (recipe below)** *or*
> **Garlic-Parmesan Coating (recipe below)**
>
> *Herbed Blue Cheese Coating*:
> **1 cup buttermilk**
> **1/4 cup crumbled blue cheese (2 oz.)**
> **1-3/4 cups dry bread crumbs**
> **1/4 teaspoon dried rosemary, crumbled**
> **1/2 teaspoon dried sage, crumbled**
> **1/2 teaspoon paprika**
> **1/4 teaspoon pepper**
>
> *Garlic-Parmesan Coating*:
> **1 cup buttermilk**
> **2 garlic cloves, pressed *or* minced**
> **1 cup dry bread crumbs**
> **1/2 cup wheat germ**
> **1/4 cup grated Parmesan cheese**
> **1/2 teaspoon dried oregano**
> **1/2 teaspoon paprika**
> **1/2 teaspoon dried thyme**
> **1/4 teaspoon pepper**

Preheat oven to 350F (175C). Line a large baking pan with foil; set aside. Prepare Herbed Blue Cheese Coating *or* Garlic-Parmesan Coating. Dip chicken pieces in buttermilk coating on all sides; roll in seasoned crumbs. With your fingers, press in crumbs. Arrange chicken pieces in baking pan so they do not touch. Bake in preheated oven for 50 minutes or until meat near thigh bone is no longer pink when slashed. Makes 6 servings.

Herbed Blue Cheese Coating:
Process buttermilk and blue cheese in a blender until smooth; pour into a shallow bowl. In another shallow bowl, combine bread crumbs, rosemary, sage, paprika and pepper.

Garlic-Parmesan Coating:
Combine buttermilk and garlic in a shallow bowl. In another shallow bowl, combine bread crumbs, wheat germ, Parmesan cheese, oregano, paprika, thyme and pepper.

PER SERVING: (Herbed Blue Cheese Coating): 1/6 of total recipe				
CALORIES	CARBOHYDRATES	PROTEIN	FAT	CHOLESTEROL
348	23 gm	32 gm	13 gm	95 mg

PER SERVING: (Garlic Parmesan Coating): 1/6 of total recipe				
CALORIES	CARBOHYDRATES	PROTEIN	FAT	CHOLESTEROL
312	18 gm	32 gm	12 gm	90 mg

Chicken-in-a-Pouch with Vegetables

On a night when you are rushed, tired, and have no interest in cooking, wrap up this convenience dinner and let the oven do the work while you take a brisk walk or just sit and relax.

> 1 chicken thigh, skin removed (5 oz.)
> 1 medium-size carrot, cut in half, each half quartered
>   lengthwise (4 oz.)
> 3 (1-inch-wide) strips green bell pepper
> 1 small potato, peeled, quartered (4 oz.)
> 1/4 teaspoon garlic salt
> Pepper to taste
> 1/8 teaspoon celery seeds
> 1/8 teaspoon paprika
> 1 tablespoon dry white wine

Preheat oven to 350F (175C). Cut a 12-inch square of heavy duty foil. In center of foil, place chicken, carrot, bell pepper and potato. Sprinkle with garlic salt, pepper to taste, celery seeds, paprika and wine. Pull up edges of foil to make a pouch; fold edges over to seal. Place pouch, sealed-side-up, in a pie pan. Bake in preheated oven for 45 minutes or until meat near thigh bone is no longer pink when slashed. Makes 1 serving.

PER SERVING: 1 serving

CALORIES	CARBOHYDRATES	PROTEIN	FAT	CHOLESTEROL
375	32 gm	34 gm	11 gm	101 mg

Chicken-in-a-Pouch with Broccoli & Mushrooms

A pouch dinner tastes better and is more economical than a frozen TV dinner. You'll have a savings in sodium too. The average commercially prepared entree runs at least 1100 milligrams of sodium per serving, compared to 626 milligrams in this oven-meal.

> 1 chicken thigh, skin removed (5 oz.)
> 1 small potato, peeled, quartered (4 oz.)
> 2 large mushrooms, cut in half
> 3 broccoli flowerets
> 1/4 teaspoon garlic salt
> 1 teaspoon olive oil
> 1 teaspoon sunflower seeds
> Pepper to taste

Preheat oven to 350F (175C). Cut a 12-inch square of heavy duty foil. In center of foil, place chicken, potato, mushrooms and broccoli. Sprinkle with garlic salt, olive oil, sunflower seeds and pepper to taste. Pull up edges of foil to make a pouch; fold edges over to seal. Place pouch, sealed-side-up, in a pie pan. Bake in preheated oven for 45 minutes or until meat near thigh bone is no longer pink when slashed. Makes 1 serving.

PER SERVING: 1 serving

CALORIES	CARBOHYDRATES	PROTEIN	FAT	CHOLESTEROL
346	26 gm	30 gm	14 gm	78 mg

Tandoori Chicken

Take a culinary passage to India with your barbecue standing in for the traditional clay tandoor oven. Because it is boned, the exotically spiced chicken cooks quickly and stays moist even without its skin. Sliced tomatoes and Puffy Broiler Bread, page 167, make fine accompaniments.

> **6 boneless chicken thighs, skin removed**
>   **(about 1-1/2 lbs.** *total***)**
> **4 garlic cloves, pressed** *or* **minced**
> **2 teaspoons grated fresh gingerroot**
> **2 tablespoon lemon juice**
> **1 tablespoon vegetable oil**
> **1 teaspoon paprika**
> **1/2 teaspoon ground coriander**
> **1/4 teaspoon ground cumin**
> **1/4 teaspoon salt**
> **1/4 teaspoon pepper**
> **1/8 teaspoon ground cinnamon**
> **1/8 teaspoon ground cloves**
> **1/8 teaspoon ground nutmeg**
> **1/8 teaspoon red (cayenne) pepper**

Place chicken in a 13" x 9" glass baking dish. In a small bowl, combine garlic, gingerroot, lemon juice, oil, paprika, coriander, cumin, salt, pepper, cinnamon, cloves, nutmeg and red pepper; mix well. Pour over chicken. With your hands, rub seasonings into chicken on all sides. Cover and refrigerate for 1 hour or up to overnight. Preheat grill or broiler; lightly grease with vegetable nonstick cooking spray. If grilling: arrange chicken on grill 4 to 6 inches above a solid bed of low-glowing coals. If broiling: arrange chicken 4 inches from heat. Cook for 4 minutes on each side or until meat in thickest part is no longer pink when slashed. Makes 6 servings.

PER SERVING: 1/6 of total recipe

CALORIES	CARBOHYDRATES	PROTEIN	FAT	CHOLESTEROL
249	0 gm	31 gm	13 gm	103 mg

Two-way Barbecued Chicken

To stay moist on the grill, this chicken needs to cook under its skin. To save time, prebaking is a good trick with bone-in chicken. It guards against meat that burns on the outside before cooking through in the middle. Here are two marinades to use with this technique.

2 broiler-fryer chickens, cut into pieces (about 3 lbs. *each*)
Gingered Fruit Baste (recipe below) *or*
Texas-Style Barbecue Sauce (recipe below)

Gingered Fruit Baste:
1/2 cup orange juice
1/2 cup apple juice
2 tablespoons packed brown sugar
1 garlic clove, pressed *or* minced
1 tablespoon lemon juice
1 tablespoon soy sauce
1/2 teaspoon ground ginger
1/2 teaspoon pepper
1 teaspoon grated orange peel

Texas-Style Barbecue Sauce:
1/2 cup dry red wine
2 tablespoons lemon juice
2 tablespoons molasses
1/4 cup ketchup
1 tablespoon Worcestershire sauce
2 garlic cloves, pressed *or* minced
2 green onions, minced, white part only
1 teaspoon pepper
1/4 teaspoon salt

Preheat oven to 350F (175C). Place chicken in 1 large or 2 medium-size baking pans that can fit in the oven at the same time. Cover tightly with foil. Bake in preheated oven for 30 minutes. Remove from oven; uncover. Let stand until cool. Prepare Gingered Fruit Baste or Texas-style Barbecue Sauce. Remove chicken pieces from pan drippings. Place in 2 plastic bags. Dividing marinade equally, pour over chicken in each bag. Seal bags; turn bags over to distribute marinade. Refrigerate for 8 hours or for up to 2 days. Preheat grill; lightly grease with vegetable nonstick cooking spray. Remove chicken from marinade with a slotted spoon; reserve marinade for basting. Arrange chicken pieces on prepared grill 4 to 6 inches above a solid bed of low-glowing coals. Cook, turning and basting frequently with marinade, for 20 to 25 minutes or until meat near thigh bone is no longer pink when slashed. Makes 10 servings.

Gingered Fruit Baste:
Combine all ingredients in a 2-cup measure; mix well. Makes 1 cup.

Texas-Style Barbecue Sauce:
Combine all ingredients in a 2-cup measure; whisk until evenly blended. Makes 1 cup.

PER SERVING: (Gingered Fruit Baste or Texas-Style Barbecue Sauce): 1/10 of total recipe

CALORIES	CARBOHYDRATES	PROTEIN	FAT	CHOLESTEROL
214	3 gm	33 gm	8 gm	98 mg

Chicken Breasts
with Hot Marmalade Sauce

The secret of this recipe is lemon juice. It "cooks" and tenderizes the chicken so you can broil it without the skin and still have moist, juicy meat. Do not marinade for more than two hours or the chicken will become tough. Just as it is with heat, too much lemon juice cooks the protein in the meat. If your plans change and you won't be home for dinner, broil the breasts and save them for lunch or dinner the next day. This dish is exceptionally low in calories. If you are a very active person, you can afford a double serving.

> **2 tablespoons lemon juice**
> **1/2 garlic clove, pressed *or* minced**
> **4 boneless, skinless chicken breast halves (1-1/4 lbs. *total*)**
> **Hot Marmalade Sauce (recipe below)**
> **1/4 teaspoon paprika**
>
> *Hot Marmalade Sauce:*
> **1/4 cup orange marmalade**
> **2 tablespoons lemon juice**
> **1-1/2 teaspoons soy sauce**
> **1/2 garlic clove, pressed *or* minced**
> **1/8 teaspoon ground ginger**

In a glass pie plate or other non-corrosive shallow pan, combine lemon juice and garlic. Place chicken in lemon juice; turn to coat all sides. Cover and let stand at room temperature for 1 hour or refrigerate up to 2 hours. Prepare Hot Marmalade Sauce; keep warm. Preheat broiler. Grease broiling pan with vegetable nonstick cooking spray. Place chicken on broiling pan; sprinkle with paprika. Broil 3 to 4 inches from heat, 2 to 3 minutes on each side or until meat is no longer pink when slashed in thickest part. Spoon sauce over each serving. Makes 4 servings.

Hot Marmalade Sauce:
In a small saucepan, combine marmalade, lemon juice, soy sauce, garlic and ginger. Heat to simmering; simmer 5 minutes or until syrupy.

PER SERVING: 1/4 of total recipe				
CALORIES	**CARBOHYDRATES**	**PROTEIN**	**FAT**	**CHOLESTEROL**
127	16 gm	12 gm	2 gm	32 mg

Chicken Breasts with Madeira Sauce

Boneless chicken breasts are an ideal choice for the cook on the run. Whether you bone the breasts yourself or buy them already boned, pull off and discard the skin. Pound the breast lightly to flatten the meat for more even cooking. Keep the cooked chicken scallops warm in a 200F oven while preparing the sauce.

> 4 boneless, skinless chicken breast halves (1-1/4 lbs. *total*)
> 2 tablespoons all-purpose flour
> Salt and pepper to taste
> 2 tablespoons margarine
> 2 green onions, minced, white part only
> 2/3 cup regular-strength beef broth
> 1/4 cup Madeira *or* port wine
> 1 teaspoon cornstarch dissolved in 2 teaspoons cold water
> 2 tablespoons chopped parsley

Space chicken breasts slightly apart between 2 sheets of wax paper; pound with a flat mallet until each is about a 3/8-inch-thick scallop. Place flour on a plate. Dredge each chicken scallop in flour; shake off excess. Season with salt and pepper to taste. In a large skillet melt margarine over medium-high heat. Add chicken pieces; cook for 2 minutes on each side or until lightly browned and meat is no longer pink when slashed in thickest part. Transfer to a platter; cover and keep warm. Add green onions to skillet; cook 1 minute. Add beef broth and wine to skillet. Cook over medium-high heat, stirring to scrape up browned bits. Cook until large bubbles break the surface and sauce is reduced by half. Stir cornstarch-water mixture once to recombine. Stirring constantly, add cornstarch mixture to skillet; cook, stirring, until sauce thickens slightly and turns clear. Pour sauce over chicken. Sprinkle with parsley. Makes 4 servings.

PER SERVING: 1/4 of total recipe				
CALORIES	CARBOHYDRATES	PROTEIN	FAT	CHOLESTEROL
343	7 gm	44 gm	12 gm	121 mg

Chicken with Grapes

Here is an easy and elegant dish that provides almost all of the body-building protein and niacin that you need for one day.

> 4 boneless, skinless chicken breast halves (1-1/4 lbs. *total*)
> 2 tablespoons all-purpose flour
> Salt and pepper to taste
> 2 tablespoons margarine
> 1/2 cup dry white wine
> 1/2 teaspoon dried tarragon
> 1 tablespoon orange marmalade
> 1-1/2 cups green seedless grapes

Space chicken breasts slightly apart between 2 sheets of wax paper; pound with a flat mallet until each is about a 3/8-inch-thick scallop. Place flour on a plate. Dredge each chicken scallop in flour; shake off excess. Season with salt and pepper to taste. In a large skillet melt margarine over medium-high heat. Add chicken pieces; cook for 2 minutes on each side or until lightly browned and meat is no longer pink when slashed in thickest part. Transfer to a platter; cover and keep warm. Add wine to skillet. Cook over medium-high heat, stirring to scrape up browned bits. Add tarragon and marmalade. Cook until large shiny bubbles appear and sauce thickens slightly. Add grapes. Cook for 1 minute to heat through. Pour sauce over chicken. Makes 4 servings.

PER SERVING: 1/4 of total recipe				
CALORIES	CARBOHYDRATES	PROTEIN	FAT	CHOLESTEROL
386	18 gm	44 gm	12 gm	117 mg

Chicken Breasts with Lemon & Capers

This is an easy, quick party dish, especially if you pound the chicken breasts ahead of time. Serve it with Broccoli-Stuffed Onions, page 147, and hot buttered pasta for a marvelous Mediterranean meal.

4 boneless, skinless chicken breast halves (1-1/4 lbs. *total*)
2 tablespoons all-purpose flour
Pepper to taste
2 tablespoons margarine
3/4 cup regular-strength chicken broth
2 tablespoons lemon juice
2 teaspoons capers, rinsed, drained
1/2 teaspoon cornstarch dissolved in 1 teaspoon cold water
1 tablespoon chopped parsley

Space chicken breasts slightly apart between 2 sheets of wax paper; pound with a flat mallet until each is about a 3/8-inch-thick scallop. Place flour on a plate. Dredge each chicken scallop in flour; shake off excess. Season with pepper to taste. In a large skillet melt margarine over medium-high heat. Add chicken pieces; cook for 2 minutes on each side or until lightly browned and meat is longer pink when slashed in thickest part. Transfer to a platter; cover and keep warm. Add chicken broth to skillet; cook over medium-high heat, stirring to scrape up browned bits. Add lemon juice and capers. Cook until bubbly. Stir cornstarch-water mixture once to recombine. Stirring constantly, add cornstarch mixture to skillet; cook, stirring, until sauce thickens slightly and turns clear. Pour sauce over chicken. Sprinkle with parsley. Makes 4 servings.

PER SERVING: 1/4 of total recipe				
CALORIES	CARBOHYDRATES	PROTEIN	FAT	CHOLESTEROL
318	5 gm	44 gm	12 gm	120 mg

Chicken & Spinach Enchiladas

For south-of-the-border flavor, here's a taste of Mexico. If time is a factor, you can make it ahead and bake it later. One enchilada makes a satisfying serving. If you've been rigorously exercising, then two enchiladas would not be out of line.

1 (10-oz.) pkg. frozen chopped spinach, thawed, drained *or*
   1 cup chopped cooked spinach
3/4 cup low-fat cottage cheese
1 (4-oz.) can diced green chiles
1/4 teaspoon dried oregano
1/4 teaspoon ground cumin
1/4 teaspoon salt
1-1/2 cups shredded cooked chicken breast
1 (19-oz.) can enchilada sauce
8 corn tortillas
1/2 cup shredded farmer cheese (2 oz.)
1/2 cup low-fat sour cream
2 green onions, sliced, including tops

With cupped hands, squeeze spinach dry; place in a medium-size bowl. Add cottage cheese, green chiles, oregano, cumin and salt; mix well. Place chicken on a plate next to spinach mixture. In a small skillet, heat half of enchilada sauce until bubbly; remove from heat. Spread a spoonful of sauce over the bottom of a 13" x 9" baking dish. To assemble each enchilada, place one tortilla in warm sauce; remove with slotted spatula and place on a plate. Place 3 tablespoons of spinach filling in center of tortilla. Cover filling with 3 tablespoons of chicken. Roll tortilla to enclose. Place seam-side-down, horizontally, in one end of baking dish. Repeat until all tortillas are filled. Pour all remaining enchilada sauce over tortillas, being sure that the ends of each tortilla are moistened. Sprinkle cheese over enchiladas. If made ahead, cover and refrigerate until next day. Preheat oven to 375F (190C). Bake covered, for 30 minutes (45 minutes if refrigerated) or until hot and bubbly. Spoon 1 tablespoon sour cream over each enchilada; sprinkle with green onion. Makes 8 enchiladas.

PER SERVING: 1 enchilada				
CALORIES	CARBOHYDRATES	PROTEIN	FAT	CHOLESTEROL
262	30 gm	19 gm	8 gm	36 mg

Stir-Fried Chicken With Vegetables

When you tumble this collection of chicken and vegetables in a wok, you add up nutrients that total, in each serving, your day's requirement for vitamins A and C plus a good amount of iron and energy-producing niacin. The exceptionally high percentage of vitamin C enables the body to utilize the iron more efficiently. Serve it with steamed rice for a quick, satisfying dinner.

> **Stir-Fry Gravy (recipe below)**
> **1 teaspoon cornstarch**
> **1 teaspoon water**
> **2 teaspoon dry sherry**
> **1/4 teaspoon salt**
> **1 large chicken breast, skinned, boned, cut in
>   bite-size pieces (1 lb.)**
> **1 tablespoon pine nuts**
> **5 teaspoons vegetable oil**
> **1 garlic clove, pressed *or* minced**
> **1 teaspoon minced fresh gingerroot**
> **1 medium-size red bell pepper, seeded, cored, cut in
>   3/4 inch squares (6 oz.)**
> **2 cups broccoli flowerets**
> **1 medium-size onion, cut in wedges, layers separated (5 oz.)**
> **1/4 cup regular-strength chicken broth *or* water**
>
> *Stir-Fry Gravy:*
> **1/2 cup water**
> **1 tablespoon cornstarch**
> **1 tablespoon soy sauce**

Prepare gravy; set aside. In small bowl, combine cornstarch, water, sherry and salt; stir to dissolve cornstarch. Add chicken; stir to coat. Let stand 15 minutes. Place a dry wok or skillet over medium heat. Add pine nuts. Stir and cook 2 minutes or until lightly toasted. Remove nuts from wok. Heat wok over high heat. When wok is hot, add 3 teaspoons of the oil. Add garlic and ginger; cook 10 seconds. Add chicken; stir-fry for 3 minutes or until chicken turns white throughout. Remove chicken from wok. Heat the remaining 2 teaspoons oil. Add bell pepper, broccoli and onion; stir-fry 30 seconds. Add chicken broth; cover pan. Cook 3 minutes or until vegetables are crisp-tender. Return chicken to wok. Stir through gravy once to recombine. Add to wok. Cook, stirring, until gravy bubbles and thickens. Stir in pine nuts. Serve immediately. Makes 3 servings.

Stir-Fry Gravy:
In a small bowl combine water, cornstarch and soy sauce; stir to dissolve cornstarch.

PER SERVING: 1/3 of total recipe				
CALORIES	CARBOHYDRATES	PROTEIN	FAT	CHOLESTEROL
345	16 gm	39 gm	14 gm	96 mg

Chicken-Mushroom Fettucini

After a long day of bicycling, satisfy your hunger in a hurry with this tasty pasta dish. It is a great source of protein, thiamin, riboflavin and niacin, and one serving gives you about twice the amount of potassium as a medium-size banana.

2 teaspoons olive oil
2 chicken thighs, boned, skinned, cut in
  1/2-inch-square pieces (10 oz.)
6 medium-size mushrooms, sliced
1 tablespoon dry white wine
1 cup Quick Tomato Sauce (page 139) *or*
  purchased marinara sauce
4 oz. whole wheat fettucini *or* regular fettucini
1 tablespoon grated Parmesan cheese

In a skillet heat oil over medium heat. Add chicken. Cook, stirring occasionally, for 4 minutes or until chicken turns opaque. Add mushrooms and wine. Cook until all liquid evaporates and mushrooms just begin to turn golden. Add Quick Tomato Sauce. Bring to a simmer over high heat. Reduce heat; simmer, uncovered, for 10 minutes. In a large kettle of boiling water, cook fettucini 8 to 10 minutes or until tender but firm to the bite; drain. Place fettucini in a serving bowl. Pour sauce over the top. Toss gently. Sprinkle with Parmesan cheese. Makes 2 servings.

PER SERVING: 1/2 of total recipe				
CALORIES	CARBOHYDRATES	PROTEIN	FAT	CHOLESTEROL
444	43 gm	32 gm	16 gm	83 mg

Rosemary-Scented Chicken Pilaf

If you are used to thinking of pilaf as a side-dish, think again. Here is one that combines lean protein and carbohydrates for an entree that's packed with vitamin C, thiamin and iron. Spinach & Apple Salad, page 151, makes a cool, crisp starter to this meal.

1 tablespoon vegetable oil
1 medium-size onion, chopped (5 oz.)
1 garlic clove, pressed *or* minced
1 medium-size green bell pepper, seeded, chopped (6 oz.)
1 lb. chicken thighs, skinned, boned, cut into 1/2-inch-square
  pieces
1 teaspoon dried rosemary, crumbled
1 cup long-grain white rice
1 large tomato, peeled, seeded, chopped (6 oz.)
1 (14-1/2-oz.) can regular-strength chicken broth *or* 1-3/4 cups
  homemade chicken broth
1/2 teaspoon salt
1/4 teaspoon pepper

In a 3-quart saucepan heat oil over medium heat. Add onion, garlic and bell pepper; cook until onion is soft but not browned. Add chicken and rosemary; cook, uncovered, for 5 minutes. Add rice; stir for 1 minute. Add tomato, chicken broth, salt and pepper; bring to a boil over high heat. Reduce heat; cover and simmer 20 minutes or until rice is tender and almost all liquid is absorbed. Makes 4 servings.

PER SERVING: 1/4 of total recipe				
CALORIES	CARBOHYDRATES	PROTEIN	FAT	CHOLESTEROL
415	46 gm	29 gm	12 gm	84 mg

Madras Chicken Buns

Move over Sloppy Joes! Here's a hearty sandwich that's quick and easy to prepare and contains very little fat, yet is loaded with lean protein.

1/4 cup low-fat sour cream
2 tablespoons mango chutney *or* other fruit chutney, chopped
1 tablespoon margarine
1/4 cup finely chopped onion
1/4 cup chopped red *or* green bell pepper
1/2 cup diced celery
1 cup coarsely chopped Granny Smith *or* other tart apple
3/4 to 1 teaspoon curry powder
1-1/2 cups diced cooked chicken breast
4 hamburger buns

In a small bowl, combine sour cream and chutney until well blended; reserve. In a skillet melt margarine over medium heat. Add onion, bell pepper, celery and apple; cook until onion is soft but not browned. Stir in curry powder; cook 1 minute. Add chicken; cook for 3 minutes or until heated through. Stir in reserved sour cream mixture; cook for 1 minute. Remove skillet from heat; keep warm. Place buns, cut side up, on a baking sheet. Preheat broiler; broil 3 inches from heat or until lightly toasted. Spoon 1/2 cup of chicken mixture onto bottom half of each bun; cover with top. Makes 4 sandwiches.

PER SERVING: 1 sandwich				
CALORIES	CARBOHYDRATES	PROTEIN	FAT	CHOLESTEROL
308	33 gm	24 gm	9 gm	56 mg

Fontina Turkey with Tomato-Basil Sauce

Mark this for summer enjoyment when fresh basil is available and tomatoes are bursting with sweetness. The recipe makes a generous amount of sauce. You might want to save out several spoonfuls, toss it with pasta and serve alongside the luscious entree.

3 medium-size tomatoes, peeled, seeded, quartered (1 lb. *total*)
1 cup packed fresh basil leaves
2 tablespoons lemon juice
1 tablespoon olive oil
Salt to taste
2 drops hot pepper sauce
1-1/2 lbs. boned turkey breast, cut in 1/4-inch-thick slices
2 tablespoons all-purpose flour
2 tablespoons margarine
24 fresh basil leaves
3 oz. Fontina cheese, thinly sliced

In a food processor, combine the tomatoes and the 1 cup of basil. Process just until tomatoes are coarsely chopped; mixture should not be pureed. Add lemon juice, olive oil and hot pepper sauce. Process 2 seconds; add salt to taste. Pour tomato-basil sauce into a serving container and set aside. Space turkey slices slightly apart between 2 sheets of wax paper; pound with a flat mallet until each is a 1/8-inch-thick scallop. Place flour on a plate. Dredge each turkey scallop in flour; shake off excess. In a large skillet melt 1 tablespoon of the margarine over medium-high heat. Add half the turkey slices. Cook for 30 seconds or until lightly browned. Turn slices over; cook for 30 more seconds or until meat is no longer pink when slashed in thickest part. Place in a single layer, in a 15" x 10" shallow baking pan; set aside. Add the remaining 1 tablespoon margarine to skillet; cook the remaining turkey. Transfer to pan; place in a single layer. Dividing them equally, place the 24 basil leaves atop turkey scallops. Cover basil with cheese. Preheat broiler. Broil 3 inches from heat until cheese melts. Pass tomato-basil sauce at the table to spoon over each serving. Makes 6 servings.

PER SERVING: 1/6 of total recipe

CALORIES	CARBOHYDRATES	PROTEIN	FAT	CHOLESTEROL
286	4 gm	37 gm	11 gm	90 mg

Turkey Scallopine with Peas

This colorful dish is a good source of niacin and fiber. It is a good dish to serve after a long race because it replaces depleted potassium. If you use ground sage instead of the whole leaf, reduce the amount to 1/2 teaspoon.

1 (8-oz.) can tomatoes
1 lb. boned turkey breast, cut in 1/4-inch-thick slices
2 tablespoons all-purpose flour
2 tablespoons margarine
1/4 cup dry white wine
1/2 cup regular-strength chicken broth
1 teaspoon dried sage, crumbled
1 (10-oz.) pkg. frozen green peas, thawed

Preheat oven to 200F (95C). Pour tomatoes and their liquid into a blender or food processor; process to make a puree; set aside. Space turkey slices slightly apart between 2 sheets of wax paper; pound with a flat mallet until each is a 1/8-inch-thick scallop. Place flour on a plate. Dredge each turkey scallop in flour; shake off excess. In a large skillet melt 1 tablespoon of the margarine over medium-high heat. Add half the turkey slices. Cook for 30 seconds or until lightly browned. Turn slices over; cook for 30 more seconds or until meat is no longer pink when slashed in thickest part. Transfer to a platter. Add the remaining 1 tablespoon margarine to skillet; cook the remaining turkey. Transfer to a platter. Cover and keep turkey warm in preheated oven. Add wine to skillet. Cook over medium-high heat, stirring to scrape up browned bits. Add pureed tomatoes, chicken broth and sage. Heat to simmering; simmer 5 minutes or until sauce thickens slightly. Add peas; cook for 1 minute to heat through. Pour sauce over turkey. Makes 4 servings.

PER SERVING: 1/4 of total recipe

CALORIES	CARBOHYDRATES	PROTEIN	FAT	CHOLESTEROL
327	16 gm	39 gm	10 gm	79 mg

Turkey Lasagne

Here's a delicious way to streamline an old standby. One serving of this creamy lasagne has less fat and fewer calories than a serving of the traditional meat and cheese variety.

3 tablespoons margarine
4-1/2 tablespoons all-purpose flour
1/4 teaspoon ground nutmeg
1/4 teaspoon white pepper
3/4 teaspoon salt
1-1/2 cups skim milk
1 cup regular-strength chicken broth
1 teaspoon lemon juice
1 (8-oz.) pkg. lasagne noodles
2 cups bite-size pieces, cooked, skinned turkey *or*
  chicken breast
1 cup shredded part-skim mozzarella cheese (4 oz.)

Crumb Topping:
2 slices French bread *or* other firm-textured bread,
  crusts removed
1 tablespoon melted margarine

In a skillet melt margarine over medium heat. Stir in flour, nutmeg, pepper and salt; cook 1 minute or until bubbly. Remove skillet from heat. Gradually stir in milk and chicken broth. Return skillet to heat. Cook, stirring, until sauce is smooth and thick. Stir in lemon juice. Remove skillet from heat; set aside. In a large kettle of boiling water, cook lasagne 10 minutes or until tender but firm to the bite. Drain, rinse with cold water and drain again. Grease a 9-inch square pan with vegetable nonstick cooking spray. Spread a thin layer of sauce over pan bottom. Cutting lasagne to fit, arrange 1/3 of noodles over sauce. Spread 1/3 of turkey over noodles. Top with 1/3 of sauce. Cover with 1/3 of cheese. Repeat this layering two more times, ending with a cheese layer. Prepare Crumb Topping. Sprinkle crumbs evenly over lasagne. If made ahead, cover and refrigerate until next day. Bake, covered, in 350F (175C) oven for 20 minutes. Uncover; continue baking for 20 more minutes (30 minutes if refrigerated) or until hot and bubbly. If crumb topping is not brown, place under preheated broiler for 10 seconds or until crumbs turn golden. Cut in squares to serve. Makes 9 servings.

Crumb Topping:
Tear bread into small chunks; drop into food processor. Process to make fine crumbs. With motor running, pour melted margarine down feed tube; process 30 seconds.

PER SERVING: 1/9 of total recipe				
CALORIES	**CARBOHYDRATES**	**PROTEIN**	**FAT**	**CHOLESTEROL**
248	20 gm	19 gm	10 gm	43 mg

FISH & SHELLFISH

Twenty years ago people would have laughed at the idea of eating fish three times a week, but not now. Fish and shellfish are now popular entrees. Food from the sea is packed with protein, niacin and potassium and has more mineral content than meat. Fish is very low in fat and easy to digest—a bonus for the athlete who wants to exercise soon after eating.

Fish is heart-healthy food. Studies indicate that certain polyunsaturated fish oils (EPA and DHA for short) can reduce triglycerides and blood cholesterol. These Omega-3 fatty acids lower the level of cholesterol in the blood, reduce the tendency of blood to form clots, and have anti-inflammatory properties beneficial for diseases such as arthritis. Fatty fish, such as salmon, mackerel, eel and herring contain more of these heart-protective fatty acids, but even lean fish may have a cholesterol lowering effect.

The bottom line is that fish is nutritious, tastes good and is very easy to cook. Fresh Catch with Herbed Yogurt Sauce, page 110, Teriyaki Fish, page 111 and Deviled Fish Kebabs, page 112, cook in minutes under the broiler or on the grill. Fettucini Veracruz, page 115, is a variation on a classic Mexican dish. Instead of frying fish and topping it with spicy Veracruz sauce, you poach the fish in the sauce, then toss it with pasta for a power-packed entree—a real savings in cooking fat and cleanup time. With a can of tuna from the pantry, you can whip up Sweet & Sour Tuna, page 120, on a moment's notice. If shrimp is your favorite, try Shrimp in the Shell, page 121; cooking these crustaceans in the shell saves preparation time, and locks in the juices during cooking.

To test fish for doneness, it is very important to cook just until the flesh is slightly opaque in the thickest part of the fish, and the flesh just starts to flake (fish separates readily at natural divisions). The fish continues to cook in its own heat as it's being served. If cooked until the fish flakes it will be overcooked and may be dry once you serve it.

Fresh Catch with Herbed Yogurt Sauce

Here is potassium-rich entree. This recipe makes a generous amount of sauce—enough to spoon over sliced tomatoes or lettuce hearts the next day.

1 cup plain low-fat yogurt
1/2 medium-size cucumber, peeled, seeded, finely
   diced (half 8 oz.)
1 small garlic clove, pressed *or* **minced**
1 teaspoon olive oil
1-1/2 teaspoons white wine vinegar
1-1/2 teaspoons minced fresh dill *or* **1/2 teaspoon dried dill**
Dash salt
2 teaspoons vegetable oil
4 firm-textured white fish fillets *or* **steaks (ling cod, sea bass,**
   red snapper *or* **halibut) about 3/4-inch thick (1-1/4 lbs.** *total***)**
Salt and pepper to taste

In a medium-size bowl, combine yogurt, cucumber, garlic, olive oil, wine vinegar, dill and a dash of salt. Cover and refrigerate for 30 minutes. Preheat broiler and broiling pan. Grease broiling pan with vegetable nonstick cooking spray. Rub vegetable oil on both sides of each fillet. Sprinkle with salt and pepper to taste. Place fillets on broiling pan. Broil 4 to 6 inches from heat for 4 minutes; turn and continue to broil 2 to 4 more minutes or until fish turns opaque and just begins to flake. Transfer fish to a platter. Pass yogurt sauce at the table to spoon over each serving. Cover and refrigerate any remaining sauce. Makes 4 servings.

PER SERVING: 1/4 of total recipe

CALORIES	CARBOHYDRATES	PROTEIN	FAT	CHOLESTEROL
329	7 gm	47 gm	12 gm	123 mg

Teriyaki Fish

Delicious grilled or broiled, fish in teriyaki sauce gives you an abundance of lean protein, niacin and calcium. For a traditional Japanese meal, serve it with unbuttered unsalted rice and stir-fried zucchini and red bell peppers. To give the rice a flavor punch, pass a bowl of wafer-thin sliced pickled ginger. It's available in Japanese markets, and once opened will keep for several months in the refrigerator.

1/4 cup soy sauce
1-1/2 tablespoons sugar
1 tablespoon dry sherry
1/4 teaspoon grated fresh gingerroot
1 small garlic clove, pressed *or* minced
1-1/2 lbs. salmon, swordfish *or* tuna steaks, 3/4 inch thick
2 teaspoons sesame seeds

In a small pan, combine soy sauce and sugar. Place over low heat until sugar dissolves. Remove from heat; let cool. Add sherry, ginger and garlic. Place fish in a plastic bag. Pour marinade over fish; seal bag. Turn bag over to distribute marinade. Refrigerate for 1 hour. Place sesame seeds in a small dry skillet. Toast over low heat, shaking skillet frequently, for 2 minutes or until seeds turn golden and begin to pop; set aside. Remove fish from marinade, drain briefly; reserve marinade for basting. Preheat broiler and broiling pan. Grease broiling pan with vegetable nonstick cooking spray. Place fish on broiling pan. Broil 4 to 6 inches from heat for 4 minutes, basting occasionally with marinade. Turn fish over. Continue to cook, basting occasionally, 2 to 4 more minutes or until fish turns opaque and just begins to flake. Remove steaks to serving plates. Sprinkle with toasted sesame seeds. Makes 4 servings.

PER SERVING: 1/4 of total recipe				
CALORIES	CARBOHYDRATES	PROTEIN	FAT	CHOLESTEROL
339	2 gm	49 gm	13 gm	84 mg

What Kind Of Soy Sauce To Use:
The flavor of soy sauce varies from brand to brand. For all purpose cooking use one of the Japanese brands widely available in supermarkets. If you are concerned about sodium, look for lite soy sauce now available in grocery stores nationwide or make your own "lite" soy by combining equal parts Japanese soy sauce and distilled water.

Deviled Fish Kebabs

Broil the kebabs if the weather is stormy, or if it's a balmy evening, you may want to cook them on the grill. Accompany with rice or noodles.

> 1/4 cup lemon juice
> 2 tablespoons vegetable oil
> 1 tablespoon sugar
> 1 tablespoon Worcestershire sauce
> 2 teaspoons Dijon-style mustard
> 1 small garlic clove, pressed *or* minced
> Salt and pepper to taste
> 1 lb. halibut *or* swordfish steaks, 1-inch thick
> 1/2 medium-size red bell pepper, cut in 1-1/2 inch
>   squares (half 6 oz.)
> 1/2 medium-size green bell pepper, cut in
>   1-1/2 inch squares (half 6 oz.)
> 1 small onion, cut in wedges, layers separated (3 oz.)

In a medium-size bowl, combine lemon juice, oil, sugar, Worcestershire, mustard, garlic and salt and pepper to taste; stir until well blended. Cut fish into 1 inch cubes; discard skin and bones. Place fish cubes in marinade; stir to coat all sides. Cover; refrigerate for 1 hour. Remove fish from marinade with a slotted spoon and drain briefly; reserve marinade for basting. On 4 (12 inch long) skewers, alternately thread fish cubes, bell pepper pieces, and onion layers. Preheat broiler and broiling pan. Grease broiling pan with vegetable nonstick cooking spray. Place skewers on broiling pan. Broil 4 to 6 inches from heat, 8 to 10 minutes, turning skewers several times and basting occasionally with marinade, until fish turns opaque and just begins to flake. Makes 4 servings.

PER SERVING: 1/4 of total recipe

CALORIES	CARBOHYDRATES	PROTEIN	FAT	CHOLESTEROL
269	8 gm	35 gm	10 gm	96 mg

Snapper Fillets au Poivre

This West coast version of blackened red fish makes a terrific dinner for two. Turn on the exhaust fan: The high heat creates smoke, but the fish stays moist and tender inside the pepper crust. To round out the meal, serve steamed broccoli and potatoes, boiled in their jackets, topped with a spoonful of cool yogurt.

> **1/4 teaspoon sea salt *or* other coarse salt**
> **1/2 teaspoon freshly ground black pepper**
> **1 tablespoon plus 1-1/2 teaspoons olive oil**
> **2 red snapper, ling cod *or* sea bass**
>   **fish fillets (5 oz. *each*)**
> **8 cherry tomatoes**
> **1 tablespoon chopped parsley**
> **1/4 teaspoon dried basil**

On a piece of wax paper, combine salt and pepper. Dredge fillets in salt-pepper mixture; coat thickly. Place a cast iron or other heavy skillet over high heat. When pan is red hot, a sprinkle of water will sizzle and evaporate. Pour in 1 tablespoon oil. Quickly tilt pan to distribute oil. Place fillets in pan. Cook 2 minutes. Turn fillets over; cook 2 more minutes or until fish turns opaque and just begins to flake. Remove pan from heat. Transfer fillets to a platter. Wipe skillet clean with paper towels. Add the remaining 1-1/2 teaspoons of oil to skillet; return skillet to high heat. Add cherry tomatoes. Swirl in skillet for 1 minute. Sprinkle with parsley and basil. Swirl tomatoes in skillet for 10 seconds. Serve parsley-coated cherry tomatoes alongside fish. Makes 2 servings.

PER SERVING: 1/2 of total recipe				
CALORIES	CARBOHYDRATES	PROTEIN	FAT	CHOLESTEROL
358	3 gm	43 gm	19 gm	120 mg

Purchasing Olive Oil:
For day to day cooking, the grades virgin olive oil and pure olive oil are very adequate and most practical in terms of cost. They are the grades used to test recipes for this book.

Oven-Fried Snapper Sticks

Pop a panful of made-at-home fish sticks into the oven for a delicious no-fuss entree. Complete the meal with Chinese Cabbage Slaw, page 152, steamed carrots, and toasted English muffins. Compared to fried fish from a fast-food restaurant, these flavorful morsels have 8 grams less fat and 14 grams more protein.

Spicy Snapper Sauce (recipe below)
1 cup seasoned Italian-style dry bread crumbs
2 tablespoons grated Parmesan cheese
1/2 teaspoon paprika
3/4 cup skim milk
1 tablespoon vegetable oil
1 1/4 lbs. boneless red snapper, orange roughy *or*
    ling cod fillets, 3/4-inch thick

Spicy Snapper Sauce:
1/4 cup ketchup
1/2 teaspoon red wine vinegar
3/4 teaspoon prepared horseradish
1/4 teaspoon Worcestershire sauce
1 tablespoon minced celery
1 teaspoon minced green onion, white part only

Prepare Spicy Snappy Sauce; set aside. Preheat oven to 450F (230C). Line a baking sheet with foil. In a pie pan, combine bread crumbs, Parmesan cheese and paprika. In a small shallow bowl, combine milk and oil. Cut fillets crosswise into 1-1/2-inch-wide pieces. Dip each piece of fish in milk mixture; dredge each piece in bread crumb mixture to thickly coat, shaking off excess. Arrange in a single layer, without crowding, on prepared baking sheet. Bake, uncovered, in preheated oven 6 to 8 minutes or until fish turns opaque and just begins to flake. Pass sauce at the table to spoon over each serving. Makes 4 servings.

Spicy Snapper Sauce:
In a small serving bowl combine ketchup, wine vinegar, horseradish, Worcestershire, celery and onion; stir until well mixed. Makes 1/3 cup.

PER SERVING: 1/4 of total recipe				
CALORIES	**CARBOHYDRATES**	**PROTEIN**	**FAT**	**CHOLESTEROL**
371	24 gm	36 gm	14 gm	93 mg

Fettucini Veracruz

For an easy Mexican-styled dinner, serve this with a salad of raw spinach, orange segments, and onion and jicama slivers tossed with Low-Cal Herb Dressing, page 162.

8 Spanish-style green olives, pitted, chopped *or*
  pimento-stuffed green olives, sliced
2 teaspoons capers
1-1/2 tablespoons olive oil
1 medium-size onion, chopped (5 oz.)
2 garlic cloves, pressed *or* minced
1 Serrano chile, seeded and minced *or* 1/4 teaspoon crushed red
  pepper flakes
1 (16-oz.) can whole peeled tomatoes
1 bay leaf
1/4 teaspoon ground cumin
1/4 teaspoon dried oregano
1/8 teaspoon pepper
1 lb. skinless red snapper, ling cod *or* orange roughy fillets,
  cut in bite-size pieces
8 oz. fettucini
2 tablespoons chopped cilantro leaves

In a sieve, separately rinse chopped olives and capers with cold water; drain on paper toweling and reserve. In a large skillet heat oil over medium heat. Add onion and garlic; cook until onion is soft but not browned. Add chile; cook 1 minute. Pour tomatoes and their liquid into skillet; coarsely cut up tomatoes. Add bay leaf, cumin, oregano, pepper and reserved olives and capers. Bring to a boil over high heat; reduce heat. Simmer, uncovered, 10 minutes. Stir in fish. Cover; simmer 10 minutes or until fish turns opaque and just begins to flake. Meanwhile, in a large kettle of boiling water, cook fettucini 8 to 10 minutes or until tender but firm to the bite; drain. Remove bay leaf from fish mixture. Place pasta in a serving bowl. Pour sauce over the top. Sprinkle with cilantro. Toss gently. Makes 4 (1-cup) servings.

PER SERVING: 1 cup				
CALORIES	CARBOHYDRATES	PROTEIN	FAT	CHOLESTEROL
396	42 gm	30 gm	12 gm	64 mg

Fish Fillets with Green Peppers

You can turn out a good dinner in a matter of minutes with a back up of frozen fish fillets. Let them thaw in the refrigerator during the day or partially defrost the block in the microwave (instructions are on the package), then cut into pieces while still frosty. Serve polenta or rice to sop up the flavorful sauce.

    1 tablespoon vegetable oil
    1 medium-size onion, cut in half, thinly sliced (5 oz.)
    1 (16-oz.) can whole peeled tomatoes
    2 medium-size green bell peppers, seeded, cored, cut in
      1/4-inch-wide strips (12 oz. *total*)
    1 teaspoon dried basil
    Salt and pepper to taste
    1 (1 lb.) pkg. frozen fish fillets (sole, perch, cod *or* haddock),
      thawed, cut in bite-size pieces
    2 tablespoons chopped parsley

In a large skillet heat oil over medium heat. Add onion; cook until soft but not browned. Pour tomatoes and their liquid into skillet; coarsely cut up tomatoes. Add bell peppers, basil and salt and pepper to taste. Cover; cook 15 minutes or until peppers are crisp-tender. Stir in fish and parsley. Simmer, uncovered, 10 to 12 minutes or until fish turns opaque and just begins to flake. Makes 4 servings.

PER SERVING: 1/4 of total recipe

CALORIES	CARBOHYDRATES	PROTEIN	FAT	CHOLESTEROL
287	12 gm	36 gm	10 gm	96 mg

Fish in Foil

Fish used to be thought of as brain food. Today's research indicates that "heart protective" is a more accurate description. Salmon in particular is high in polyunsaturated fish oils that help lower the level of blood cholesterol and reduce the tendency of blood to form clots.

    1/2 cup plain low-fat yogurt
    2 teaspoons cornstarch
    1-1/4 lbs. skinned salmon, red snapper *or* cod fillets, cut in 4
      serving pieces
    1 cup chopped, seeded tomato
    1/2 cup minced green pepper
    1/2 cup chopped onion
    1/2 teaspoon grated lemon peel
    1 small Serrano chile, seeded, minced (optional)
    Salt and pepper to taste
    1 lemon, cut in quarters
    Fresh cilantro sprigs

Cut 4 pieces of foil, each 3 times as wide and 1-1/2 times as long as fish pieces; set aside. In a bowl, combine yogurt and cornstarch; whisk until no lumps remain. Place fish in yogurt; turn to coat all sides. Let stand, covered, at room temperature for 30 minutes. Preheat oven to 425F (220C). In another bowl, combine tomato, green pepper, onion, lemon peel and chile, if used. Place 1 portion of fish in center of foil. Sprinkle with salt and pepper to taste. Spoon 1/4 of tomato mixture over fish. Bring long sides of foil together; fold to seal, then double-fold ends. Repeat with remaining fish and vegetables. Place packets, sealed-side-up, slightly apart, in a shallow rimmed baking pan. Bake in preheated oven 8 to 10 minutes or until fish turns opaque and just begins to flake. Place packet on 4 serving plates. Open each packet. Garnish with one or two cilantro sprigs and squeeze a lemon wedge over each fish serving. Makes 4 servings.

PER SERVING: 1 packet				
CALORIES	CARBOHYDRATES	PROTEIN	FAT	CHOLESTEROL
323	10 gm	44 gm	11 gm	71 mg

Poached Salmon with Sauce Verte

Here's a lean dish fresh from your own kitchen. One serving of this niacin-rich entree supplies 60% of the US RDA for protein, yet has less fat than 2 tablespoons of peanut butter. If the weather is hot, you can poach the fish a day ahead and serve it chilled. Or for a wintry meal, serve it hot with boiled thin-skinned potatoes.

1/3 cup cooked spinach, chopped, drained (8 oz. fresh)
1/3 cup low-fat sour cream
1/3 cup plain low-fat yogurt
1 tablespoon chopped parsley
2 teaspoons minced green onion, white part only
1/4 teaspoon dried dill
2 drops hot pepper sauce
Salt to taste
1-1/2 lbs. salmon fillet or steaks, poached, page 118
Watercress or parsley sprigs

With cupped hands, squeeze spinach dry. Drop in food processor or blender. Add sour cream, yogurt, parsley, green onion, dill and hot pepper sauce; process until sauce is smooth and bright green. Add salt to taste. Pour into a serving bowl; cover and refrigerate for 2 hours or up to 2 days. Meanwhile poach fish; remove skin and bones. Serve warm or cover and refrigerate for up to 24 hours. Arrange fish on a serving platter. Garnish with watercress. Pass sauce at the table to spoon over each serving. Makes 6 servings.

PER SERVING: 1/6 of total recipe				
CALORIES	CARBOHYDRATES	PROTEIN	FAT	CHOLESTEROL
236	2 gm	34 gm	9 gm	58 mg

Poached Fish

Since no fat is used in poaching, fish cooked by this technique tastes best when it simmers in a seasoned broth called court bouillon. Use this all-purpose broth any time you want to serve hot or chilled poached fish or when you want cooked fish to use in a salad, casserole, or as a sandwich filling. One pound of boneless fish yields 2 cups of cooked fish. If you need a very large quantity of fish, double the poaching broth; just be sure there is enough liquid to cover the fish. To estimate poaching time, lay fish a on flat surface and measure height of thickest portion. Follow instructions in recipe for poaching time.

        4 cups water
        1 small onion, sliced (3 oz.)
        6 whole black peppercorns
        3 whole allspice
        1 bay leaf
        2 parsley sprigs
        2 tablespoons lemon juice
        1/2 cup dry white wine
        2 to 3 lbs. fish fillets, steaks *or* whole cleaned fish

In a large kettle, combine water, onion, peppercorns, allspice, bay leaf, parsley, lemon juice and wine. Bring to a boil over high heat; reduce heat. Cover and simmer 30 minutes. Add fish; cover and simmer over low heat until fish turns opaque and just begins to flake. As a rule of thumb count on 10 minutes of cooking per inch of thickness; a 1/2-inch-thick fillet will cook in 5 minutes; a 1-inch-thick fillet will cook in 10 minutes; a 1-1/2-inch-thick fillet or steak or whole fish 1-1/2-inches thick will cook in about 15 minutes. With a wide slotted spatula, remove fish from poaching broth to a rimmed plate; discard poaching broth. Serve hot, or if served cold, let cool; cover and refrigerate for up to 2 days.

Nutritional data for this basic recipe is not included because the particular type and amount of fish a person should cook or eat is not specified. Other recipes in this chapter, which specify type and amount of fish to be poached include nutritional data.

Filet of Sole Martini

Pick up the makings of this entree on the way home from your workout; you can assemble it in minutes. The sauce is light and so good you'll want to serve rice or bulgur to soak up every bit of its flavorful sauce.

> 1 (6-oz.) can vegetable cocktail juice
> 1 tablespoon dry vermouth *or* dry white wine
> 1 tablespoon chopped parsley
> 1 garlic clove, pressed *or* minced
> 1 lb. skinless, sole *or* flounder fillets, about
>   1/2-inch thick
> Salt and white pepper to taste
> 1/4 lb. tiny, shelled, cooked shrimp

Preheat oven to 325F (165C). In a small bowl, combine cocktail juice, vermouth, parsley and garlic; set aside. Season fillets with salt and pepper to taste. Arrange half of fillets in a 1-quart casserole or divide evenly among 4 individual ramekins. Sprinkle with half of the shrimp. Spoon over half of cocktail mixture. Repeat layers ending with cocktail mixture. Bake, uncovered, in preheated oven for 20 minutes or until fish turns opaque and just begins to flake. Makes 4 servings.

PER SERVING: 1/4 of total recipe

CALORIES	CARBOHYDRATES	PROTEIN	FAT	CHOLESTEROL
280	2 gm	42 gm	10 gm	152 mg

Hakone Trout

One trout supplies 86% of the US RDA for protein, yet contains less fat than 3 large black olives. If you can't find boned trout, take a tip from Japanese home cooks and filet the fish on one side only. After broiling, you can easily lift off the backbone without tearing the meat.

> 1 large orange (8 oz.)
> 1/2 teaspoon grated fresh gingerroot
> 1 teaspoon soy sauce
> 2 trout, preferably boned (8 oz. *each*)
> 1/4 teaspoon salt

Cut orange in half crosswise; ream juice and pulp into a small bowl. Add ginger and soy sauce. Divide sauce between two small dipping sauce bowls; set aside. To bone trout, use a knife with a flexible blade to cut off fillet on one side of each trout. Starting at tail end, slide knife along backbone, cutting toward the head. Lift fillet as you cut; cut off from body and set aside. Cut off fish heads, if desired. Place fish halves, skin-side-down, on a baking sheet. Sprinkle fish evenly with salt. Let stand 20 minutes. Rinse fish in cold water to remove salt. Pat dry with paper towels. Preheat broiler and broiling pan. Grease broiling pan with vegetable nonstick cooking spray. Place fish halves, skin-side-down, on broiling pan. Broil 4 to 6 inches from heat, 4 to 6 minutes or until fish turns opaque and just begins to flake. Lift off back bones from unboned trout halves. Transfer fish to 2 serving plates. Serve with dipping sauce. Makes 2 servings.

PER SERVING: 1 trout

CALORIES	CARBOHYDRATES	PROTEIN	FAT	CHOLESTEROL
303	15 gm	47 gm	5 gm	117 mg

Sweet & Sour Tuna

Fish and rice are a good combination, especially satisfying after a long bicycle ride. This full-meal entree will replace your depleted glycogen and potassium levels. One serving is 88% carbohydrate and has more potassium than 10 ounces of orange juice.

1 (8-oz.) can pineapple chunks packed in juice
3 tablespoons sugar
3 tablespoons distilled white vinegar
1 teaspoon soy sauce
1/4 teaspoon dry mustard
2 tablespoons ketchup
2 tablespoons water
1-1/2 tablespoons cornstarch
1 tablespoon margarine
1 small onion, cut in quarters, thinly sliced (3 oz.)
1/2 small green bell pepper, seeded, cut in
  1-inch chunks (half 4 oz.)
1 (6-1/2-oz.) can water-pack tuna, drained,
  broken in chunks
6 cherry tomatoes, cut in half
3 cups hot cooked long-grain rice (1 cup uncooked)
1 green onion, thinly sliced, including top

Drain pineapple juice into a small bowl; reserve pineapple. Combine juice with sugar, white vinegar, soy sauce, mustard, ketchup, water and cornstarch; whisk until evenly blended then set aside. In a skillet melt margarine over medium heat. Add onion and bell pepper; cook until onion is soft but not browned. Stir pineapple juice mixture to recombine; pour into skillet. Stirring constantly, cook until sauce bubbles and thickens slightly. Add pineapple chunks, tuna and cherry tomatoes. Cook 1 minute or until heated through. Divide rice onto 3 plates. Evenly divide tuna mixture over rice. Garnish each serving with green onion. Makes 3 servings.

PER SERVING: 1/3 of total recipe

CALORIES	CARBOHYDRATES	PROTEIN	FAT	CHOLESTEROL
501	88 gm	25 gm	5 gm	42 mg

Burritos de Pescado

Each person can assemble his own eat-out-of hand entree. One serving contains 125 fewer calories and 32% less fat than a combination burrito at a Mexican fast food restaurant. Accompany with fresh fruit of the season.

Avocado Salsa (recipe opposite)
2 cups poached fish such as salmon, red snapper, turbot, *or*
  cod, (page 118), skin and bones removed, flaked
1-1/2 cups shredded iceberg lettuce
1 cup low-fat sour cream
8 (8-inch) flour tortillas

Avocado Salsa:
2 medium-size tomatoes, peeled, seeded, chopped (10 oz. *total***)**
1/4 cup chopped canned green chiles
1 green onion, thinly sliced, including top
1 medium-size avocado, halved, pitted, peeled, diced (6 oz.)
2 teaspoons lemon juice
1 tablespoon chopped cilantro leaves
Salt and pepper to taste

Prepare Avocado Salsa; set aside. Place fish, lettuce, and sour cream in individual bowls. Just before serving, preheat oven to 350F (165C). Remove paper separators, stack and wrap tortillas in foil. Heat in oven 15 minutes. Place tortillas in a basket and keep warm. Set all ingredients on the table. To assemble: Fill one tortilla with about 3 tablespoons lettuce, 1/4 cup fish, 3 tablespoons Avocado Salsa and 2 tablespoons sour cream. Roll the tortilla around the filling; eat out of hand. Makes 8 burritos.

Avocado Salsa:
In a bowl, combine tomatoes, chiles, green onion, avocado, lemon juice, cilantro and salt and pepper to taste. If made ahead, cover and refrigerate up to 4 hours.

PER SERVING: 1 burrito

CALORIES	CARBOHYDRATES	PROTEIN	FAT	CHOLESTEROL
279	22 gm	22 gm	11 gm	58 mg

Shrimp in the Shell

Dig in! There's no subtle way to eat these shrimp but by hand. Start by sucking the juices from the shrimp shell then peel, open and devour the succulent meat inside. Tossed green salad, teamed with corn on the cob and frozen juice bars, makes a fabulous meal that you can cook in less than 30 minutes.

1 lb. medium-size raw shrimp in the shell
1/8 teaspoon salt
2 tablespoons vegetable oil
2 garlic cloves, pressed *or* **minced**
1 teaspoon minced fresh gingerroot
1/8 to 1/4 teaspoon crushed red pepper (optional)
3 tablespoons dry sherry
1 tablespoon soy sauce
4 green onions, thinly sliced, including tops

With kitchen scissors, cut shrimp through backs of shells just to vein; rinse out sand vein. Pat shrimp dry with paper towels. Sprinkle salt evenly over shrimp. In a large skillet heat oil over medium-high heat. When oil is hot, add garlic and ginger; stir for 3 seconds. Add shrimp and red pepper, if used. Stir-fry for 2 minutes or just until shrimp shells turn pink. Add sherry and soy sauce; stir for 30 seconds. Add green onions; cook for 30 seconds. Serve immediately. Makes 3 servings.

PER SERVING: 1/3 of total recipe

CALORIES	CARBOHYDRATES	PROTEIN	FAT	CHOLESTEROL
207	4 gm	21 gm	10 gm	169 mg

Shrimp Istanbul

Not only does this elegant entree have less fat than one ballpark frank, it is just about as fast to cook. For a springtime company dinner, serve it with Asparagus Milanese, page 142 and rice. Serve Strawberry Sorbet, page 179, tucked in an Almond Cookie Shell, page 184, for a fantastic finale.

> **1-1/2 tablespoons margarine**
> **1 small onion, finely chopped (3 oz.)**
> **1 garlic clove, pressed *or* minced**
> **1 lb. medium-size raw shrimp, shelled, deveined**
> **1/2 cup dry white wine**
> **1 bay leaf**
> **4 medium-size tomatoes, peeled, chopped (1 lb. *total*) *or***
> **   1 (16 oz.) can whole peeled tomatoes, undrained, chopped**
> **1/2 cup water**
> **Salt and pepper to taste**
> **1/2 cup shredded farmer cheese (2 oz.)**

In a wide skillet melt margarine over medium-high heat. Add onion and garlic; cook until onion is soft but not browned. Add shrimp; cook 1 minute. Add wine and bay leaf. Cook 1 minute. Add tomatoes and water. Heat until simmering; reduce heat, cover, and simmer 4 minutes. With a slotted spoon, remove shrimp to a 1-quart ovenproof casserole; set aside. Cook sauce on high, uncovered, for 3 minutes or until sauce has thickened and most of liquid has been reduced. Discard bay leaf. Add salt and pepper to taste. Evenly spoon sauce over shrimp. Evenly sprinkle cheese over sauce. Preheat broiler. Place casserole 6 inches below broiler; broil 2 minutes or until cheese melts. Makes 4 servings.

PER SERVING: 1/4 of total recipe				
CALORIES	CARBOHYDRATES	PROTEIN	FAT	CHOLESTEROL
249	12 gm	27 gm	8 gm	188 mg

Quick Curried Scallops

In trendy restaurants, scallops, paired with pilaf, often star as a house special. No wonder—they taste superb and are good candidates for short-order cooking. Scallops are high in potassium, a low-fat source of protein, and they supply a substantial amount of iron, an important oxygen-transporting nutrient.

> **1 lb. scallops**
> **2 tablespoons margarine**
> **1 medium-size onion, cut in half, thinly sliced (5 oz.)**
> **1 large Granny Smith *or* other tart apple, quartered, cored,**
> **   peeled, thinly sliced (8 oz.)**
> **1 teaspoon curry powder**
> **1/2 cup dry white wine**
> **3 tablespoons chopped parsley**
> **Salt to taste**

If using large sea scallops, cut in halves or thirds; leave bay scallops whole. In a skillet melt margarine over medium-high heat. Add scallops; cook 2 minutes or until scallops become opaque. Remove scallops with a slotted spoon; set aside. Add onion and apple to skillet; cook 4 minutes or until onion is crisp-tender. Add curry powder; cook 30 seconds. Add wine and parsley; cook for 2 minutes or until wine is reduced by half. Add salt to taste. Return scallops to skillet. Heat through for 30 seconds. Makes 4 servings.

PER SERVING: 1/4 of total recipe

CALORIES	CARBOHYDRATES	PROTEIN	FAT	CHOLESTEROL
281	22 gm	29 gm	7 gm	63 mg

Pasta Shells with Crab & Mushrooms

Launch a weekend of cross country skiing—or any sport that calls for endurance—with a Friday night supper that tastes superb and is loaded with complex carbohydrates. With this creamy entree, you maximize energy and minimize fat: There's less fat than the equivalent of 1 tablespoon of margarine.

2 tablespoons margarine
1 tablespoon minced green bell pepper
1 tablespoon minced red bell pepper
1 cup sliced mushrooms (3 oz.)
2 tablespoons all-purpose flour
2 cups low-fat milk
1 tablespoon dry sherry
1/4 teaspoon ground nutmeg
1/3 lb. crabmeat *or* surimi-style (imitation) crabmeat
Salt and red (cayenne) pepper to taste
8-oz. medium-size pasta shells *or* other medium-size, fancy
　　shaped pasta

In a medium-size saucepan, melt margarine over medium heat. Add green and red bell pepper and mushrooms; cook until mushrooms are soft. Stir in flour; cook 1 minute or until bubbly. Remove from heat. Gradually stir in milk. Return pan to heat. Cook, stirring, until sauce comes to a boil and is the consistency of heavy cream. Stir in sherry, nutmeg and crabmeat. Add salt and red pepper to taste. Reduce heat to low; cover and keep warm. In a large kettle of boiling water, cook pasta 8 to 10 minutes or until tender but firm to the bite; drain. Place in a serving bowl. Add sauce. Toss to coat pasta. Makes 4 (1-1/3 cup) servings.

PER SERVING: 1-1/3 cups

CALORIES	CARBOHYDRATES	PROTEIN	FAT	CHOLESTEROL
343	43 gm	19 gm	10 gm	60 mg

Fisherman's Spaghetti

Tender crabmeat is combined with a tangy vegetable-ladened tomato sauce in this quick entree. One serving supplies 96% of the US RDA for vitamin C and 45% of the US RDA for vitamin A. This is a great dish to eat the night before a day of cross-country skiing.

> 2 tablespoons olive oil
> 1 medium-size onion, chopped (5 oz.)
> 1/2 cup minced celery
> 1/2 cup chopped red *or* green bell pepper
> 1 garlic clove, pressed *or* minced
> 1 (16-oz.) can whole peeled tomatoes
> 1 (8-oz.) can tomato sauce
> 1/2 cup dry white wine
> 1/2 cup water
> 1 teaspoon dried basil
> 1/4 teaspoon dried thyme
> 1/4 teaspoon dried sage
> 3 drops hot pepper sauce
> 1/2 lb. crabmeat *or* surimi-style (imitation) crabmeat, flaked, *or*
>   1/2 pound scallops
> Salt and pepper to taste
> 12 oz. spaghetti
> 2 tablespoons chopped parsley

In a large skillet heat oil over medium heat. Add onion, celery, bell pepper and garlic; cook until onion is soft but not browned. Pour tomatoes and their liquid into skillet; coarsely cut up tomatoes. Add tomato sauce, wine, water, basil, thyme, sage and hot pepper sauce. Bring to a boil over high heat; reduce heat. Simmer, uncovered, for 20 minutes or until sauce has thickened slightly. Stir in crabmeat; heat through. (If using scallops, cut large sea scallops into halves or thirds; leave bay scallops whole. Add scallops; cook 2 minutes or until scallops become opaque.) Add salt and pepper to taste; keep warm. In a large kettle of boiling water, cook spaghetti 8 to 10 minutes or until tender but firm to the bite; drain. Place in a serving bowl. Add sauce. Toss to coat pasta. Sprinkle with parsley. Makes 6 (1-1/2-cup) servings.

PER SERVING: 1-1/2 cups				
CALORIES	CARBOHYDRATES	PROTEIN	FAT	CHOLESTEROL
296	43 gm	14 gm	6 gm	38 mg

Linguini with Clam Sauce

This entree is easy and elegant—something you may order when you go out—but just as simple and leaner to make at home. A 1 cup serving provides over 100% of the US RDA for Vitamin B_{12}, a difficult nutrient to obtain when meat is excluded from the diet. Use for carbo-loading before a race.

1/2 cup chopped parsley
1 large garlic clove, pressed *or* minced
2 teaspoons grated lemon peel
2 tablespoons olive oil
1 tablespoon margarine
2 green onions, minced, white part only
2 (6-1/2 oz. *each*) cans chopped *or* minced clams
1/2 cup dry white wine
8 oz. linguini
Freshly ground black pepper to taste

In a small bowl, combine parsley, garlic and lemon peel; mix evenly. In a medium-size saucepan, heat oil and margarine over low heat. Add onions and cook until soft but not browned. Drain clam liquid into pan; reserve clams. Add wine to pan. Simmer 5 minutes or until sauce is reduced by 1/3. Add clams and 2/3 of the parsley mixture; reduce heat, cover and keep warm. (*Do not allow to boil,* or clams will be tough.) In a large kettle of boiling water, cook linguini 8 to 10 minutes or until tender but firm to the bite; drain. Place in a serving bowl. Add sauce and the remaining 1/3 of parsley mixture. Toss to coat pasta. Add pepper to taste; toss again. Makes 4 (1-cup) servings.

PER SERVING: 1 cup				
CALORIES	CARBOHYDRATES	PROTEIN	FAT	CHOLESTEROL
367	36 gm	21 gm	13 gm	68 mg

Mussels Mariner's Style

With less fat than 3 tablespoons of peanuts, one serving of this meal-in-a-bowl contributes over 100% of the US RDA for protein and a high amount of complex carbohydrates. For an easy meal, offer Spicy Poached Pears, page 178, for dessert.

    3 lbs. mussels
    1 tablespoon olive oil
    1 medium-size onion, finely chopped (5 oz.)
    1 small celery stalk with leaves, finely chopped
    1-1/2 cups dry white wine
    1/3 cup chopped parsley
    1/4 teaspoon dried thyme
    1/8 teaspoon freshly ground black pepper
    3 cups hot cooked long-grain rice (1 cup uncooked)
    1 cup canned whole peeled tomatoes, drained, chopped (8 oz.)

Scrub mussels with a brush to remove sand from shells; rinse well in cold tap water. Remove beards. Discard any mussels whose shells do not close when tapped. In a large kettle heat oil over medium heat. Add onion and celery; cook until onion is soft but not browned. Add wine, 1/2 of the parsley, thyme and pepper. Heat until liquid barely simmers. Cover; simmer 5 minutes. Add mussels. Cover; simmer 2 minutes. Stir with a large spoon so mussels cook evenly. Cook 2 to 6 more minutes or until shells open. Evenly divide rice into 4 wide bowls. Use a slotted spoon to remove cooked mussels and arrange over rice; discard any mussels that do not open. Add remaining parsley and tomatoes to broth. Heat to simmering. Ladle broth over mussels. Makes 4 servings.

PER SERVING: 1/4 of total recipe				
CALORIES	**CARBOHYDRATES**	**PROTEIN**	**FAT**	**CHOLESTEROL**
599	57 gm	57 gm	12 gm	180 mg

PIZZA, PASTA, GRAINS & SAUCES

Just as a car needs the right fuel to reach peak performance, so does your body. The body works more efficiently when at least 50% of the total calories comes from complex carbohydrates such as bread, beans, pasta, potatoes and rice.

In their natural state, these starches are not fattening. When we add butter, sour cream and cheese, they become laden with fat and are no longer fitness foods. Recipes in this chapter add flavor without fat.

Decreasing fat does not mean decreasing flavor. Try Broccoli-Stuffed Ricotta Shells, page 131, or Eggplant Lasagne, page 133, for a lively taste of Italy. Zucchini-Rice Quiche, page 134, tastes marvelous and is nutritious. Because carbohydrates are important for good health and bring great eating pleasure, they appear in other chapters of this book too. Check the index for recipes listed under beans, pasta and rice.

COOKING THE CARBOHYDRATES

When you cook pasta or rice, don't add salt to the cooking water. Pasta and rice don't need salt because they are eaten with food which is already seasoned. Contrary to old cooking myths, you don't need to add oil to the cooking water for pasta. To prevent pasta from sticking, stir to separate after adding it to the boiling water. To prevent the water from boiling over, make sure you use a kettle large enough to allow the water to boil; do not cover.

Calzone & Pizza Dough

This recipe makes enough dough for 6 large calzones or 2 (12-inch) pizzas.

1/4 cup warm water (110F/45C)
1 (1/4-oz.) pkg. active dry yeast (*about* 1 tablespoon)
3 cups all-purpose flour
1 teaspoon salt
1 teaspoon dried basil
1 teaspoon dried oregano
3/4 cup cool water
1 tablespoon honey
2 tablespoons olive oil
1 teaspoon vegetable oil

Pour warm water into a small bowl; sprinkle yeast over water and stir until dissolved. Let stand 10 minutes or until small bubbles form. In a food processor, combine flour, salt, basil and oregano; process 10 seconds. In a 1-cup glass measure, combine cool water, honey and olive oil. With food processor running, pour honey mixture down the feed tube then pour dissolved yeast down the feed tube. Process until mixture forms a ball. On a lightly floured surface, knead dough 5 minutes or until smooth and elastic.

Grease a large bowl with vegetable oil. Place dough in bowl; turn to coat. Cover bowl with a dry cloth towel; let rise in a warm, draft-free place for 1 hour or until dough doubles in bulk. Proceed with calzone or pizza recipe.

To make dough by hand:
Combine dry ingredients in a large bowl. Make a well in the center; add honey mixture and dissolved yeast. Stir with a heavy wooden spoon until dough forms. On a lightly floured surface, knead dough 10 minutes or until smooth and elastic. Proceed with instructions above for rising.

Analysis is included with each pizza or calzone recipe.

Sausage & Vegetable Pizzas

It's easy to make your own lean sausage at home, but you must wait 24 hours for flavors to blend before you use it. Try it in pizza; another time make sausage into patties for a leisurely weekend brunch. Pizza is a good choice for carbohydrate-loading before a race.

Home-Made Sausage (recipe below)
1 recipe Calzone & Pizza Dough (opposite)
1 cup Marinara Sauce (page 138) *or* **purchased marinara sauce**
2 cups shredded part-skim mozzarella cheese (8 oz.)
1/2 cup chopped onion
1 cup chopped green *or* **red bell pepper**
1 cup sliced mushrooms
1 small zucchini, thinly sliced (4 oz.)

Home-Made Sausage:
1 lb. lean ground beef *or* **lean ground pork**
1 teaspoon fennel seeds, crushed
1/2 teaspoon dried oregano
1 teaspoon dried basil
3/4 teaspoon salt
2 garlic cloves, pressed *or* **minced**

Prepare Home-Made Sausage. Prepare dough as directed on opposite page. While dough is rising, heat skillet over medium-high heat. Crumble sausage into skillet; cook until browned. Discard drippings. Let sausage cool. After dough has doubled in bulk, punch down. Let rest 10 minutes. Preheat oven to 450F (230C). Grease 2 (12-inch) pizza pans with vegetable nonstick cooking spray. Divide dough in half. Roll out each half on a lightly floured surface to a 12-inch circle. Lift dough into pans; pat firmly into pan edges. For each pizza, evenly spread half of marinara sauce over dough, leaving about 1 inch of dough uncoated at edge. Sprinkle half of cheese over sauce. Top with half of onion, bell pepper, mushrooms and zucchini. Scatter half of sausage over vegetables. Bake in preheated oven 15 to 18 minutes or until cheese melts and bottom of crust is browned. Makes 2 (12-inch) pizzas.

Home-Made Sausage:
In a bowl combine beef, fennel, oregano, basil, salt and garlic. Mix with your hands until thoroughly blended; cover. Refrigerate 24 hours to allow flavors to blend.

PER SERVING: 1/4 of 1 (12-inch) pizza				
CALORIES	CARBOHYDRATES	PROTEIN	FAT	CHOLESTEROL
454	56 gm	31 gm	15 gm	68 mg

Rose's Mixed Greens & Cheese Calzone

Here's an innovative stuffed dough treat made with Middle Eastern-spiced Swiss chard and cheese. Another time, try the tofu variation. You can serve either calzone hot or at room temperature. Enjoy it at home or slip it into a day pack to take on a hike or bike ride. Each calzone is packed with iron and vitamins A and C.

       1 recipe Calzone & Pizza Dough (page 128)
       1 lb. Swiss chard
       4 large leeks, (2 inches in diameter)
       2 tablespoons olive oil
       1 large garlic clove, pressed *or* minced
       1/2 cup chopped parsley
       1/2 teaspoon dried mint, crumbled
       1/8 teaspoon ground cinnamon
       1/4 teaspoon pepper
       1/2 teaspoon salt
       1 cup shredded Swiss cheese (4 oz.)
       2 tablespoons cornmeal

Prepare dough as directed on page 128. While dough is rising, cut off heavy chard stems; finely chop. Coarsely chop chard leaves. Reserve stems and leaves in separate bowls. Trim root ends of leeks then trim tops, leaving about 1-1/2 inches of dark green leaves. Split leeks lengthwise; rinse well. Thinly slice crosswise. Heat oil in a 5-quart kettle over medium heat. Add chard stems, leeks and garlic; cook 10 minutes. Add chard leaves, parsley, mint, cinnamon, pepper and salt; stir to mix well. Cover and cook 10 minutes or until greens are tender; uncover. Continue to cook until all liquid has evaporated; let cool. Stir cheese into cooled filling.

     After dough has doubled in bulk, punch down. Let rest 10 minutes. Preheat oven to 450F (230C). Grease 2 baking sheets with vegetable nonstick cooking spray; sprinkle with cornmeal. Divide dough into 6 equal-size pieces. Use 1 piece at a time; cover remaining pieces so they don't dry out. To make calzone, on a lightly floured board, roll each piece into a 7-inch circle. Place 1/2-cup of the filling on half of the circle, 1-inch from edge. Moisten edges of dough with water; fold uncovered half of dough over filling to make a half circle. Lightly press edges together. Fold edges of dough up onto itself to form a curl; as you curl, pinch edges to seal. Place on prepared pans. Bake in preheated oven 10 to 12 minutes or until golden brown. Serve hot or at room temperature. Makes 6 calzone.

Variation
Rose's Mixed Greens & Tofu Calzone:
Increase salt to 3/4 teaspoon. Omit cheese. Add 8-oz. regular or firm tofu, drained and patted dry. Finely crumble tofu into cooled vegetable mixture.

PER SERVING: 1 calzone with cheese				
CALORIES	**CARBOHYDRATES**	**PROTEIN**	**FAT**	**CHOLESTEROL**
427	58 gm	15 gm	15 gm	17 mg

PER SERVING: 1 calzone with tofu				
CALORIES	**CARBOHYDRATES**	**PROTEIN**	**FAT**	**CHOLESTEROL**
396	59 gm	13 gm	12 gm	0 mg

Broccoli-Stuffed Ricotta Shells

As long as it tastes good, Italian cooks will stuff pasta with just about anything. When the choice is broccoli, you gain vitamin A, potassium, iron, calcium, niacin and fiber. Serve broccoli frequently if you seldom eat meat; one cup contains 5 grams of protein.

4 cups Marinara Sauce (page 138) *or* purchased
   marinara sauce
6 cups coarsely chopped broccoli flowerets, and
   sliced, peeled stems (1-1/2 lbs.)
2 teaspoons margarine
1 small onion, chopped (3 oz.)
1 garlic clove, pressed *or* minced
2 cups part-skim ricotta cheese (16 oz.)
2 eggs
1/2 teaspoon salt
1/4 teaspoon white pepper
1/2 teaspoon dried rosemary, crumbled
1/4 teaspoon ground nutmeg
28 jumbo pasta shells (7 oz. *total*)

Prepare sauce. In a large saucepan, cook broccoli in 1 inch of boiling water 8 to 10 minutes or until tender; drain. Finely chop broccoli in a food processor or with a heavy knife; set aside. In a small skillet melt margarine over medium heat. Add onion and garlic; cook until onion is soft but not browned. Remove from heat; cool. In a large bowl, stir ricotta cheese and eggs together until well blended. Add salt, white pepper, rosemary, nutmeg, onion mixture and chopped broccoli; mix well. In a large kettle of boiling water, cook pasta shells 8 to 10 minutes or until tender but firm to the bite; stir several times while pasta is cooking to separate shells. Drain, rinse with cold water and drain again. Stuff each shell with 2-1/2 tablespoons of broccoli-cheese mixture. Pour half of the sauce into a 13″ x 9″ baking pan. Arrange filled shells in sauce. Spoon remaining sauce over the top. If assembled ahead, cover and refrigerate until next day. Preheat oven to 350F (175C). Bake, covered, 30 minutes (45 minutes if refrigerated) or until hot and bubbly. Makes 7 servings.

PER SERVING: 4 stuffed shells				
CALORIES	CARBOHYDRATES	PROTEIN	FAT	CHOLESTEROL
304	34 gm	15 gm	12 gm	92 mg

Tip:
For made-at-home convenience food, freeze unbaked stuffed shells in individual ovenproof freezer containers. Place 4 stuffed shells in each container; cover with 1/2 cup marinara sauce. Cover, label and freeze. To heat: Bake, covered, 45 minutes in a 375F (190C) oven.

Pasta with All-Seasons Pesto

Pesto is the marvelous invention of Genovese cooks. Usually made in summer when fresh basil is plentiful, this nutritious spinach pesto can be made year round. Serve this high-carbohydrate side dish with broiled fish or grilled flank steak. If you are cooking for one, allow 3 tablespoons of pesto for each cup of cooked pasta.

        1/2 cup low-fat sour cream
        1/2 cup packed spinach leaves
        1/4 cup packed parsley sprigs
        1 tablespoon dried basil
        1 small garlic clove
        2 tablespoons grated Parmesan cheese
        Salt to taste
        8 oz. fettucini *or* linguini

In a blender or food processor, combine sour cream, spinach, parsley, basil, garlic and Parmesan cheese; process until smooth. Add salt to taste. In a large kettle of boiling water, cook fettucini 8 to 10 minutes or until tender but firm to the bite; drain. Place in a serving bowl. Add sauce. Toss until pasta is well coated with sauce. Makes 4 (1-cup) servings.

PER SERVING: 1 cup

CALORIES	CARBOHYDRATES	PROTEIN	FAT	CHOLESTEROL
238	40 gm	10 gm	4 gm	56 mg

Linguini with Artichoke Sauce

In the time it takes to cook pasta, you can prepare this sauce. High in carbohydrates, it's a good choice to replace depleted glycogen and potassium after a long cross-country ski outing. One serving supplies more potassium than 1 cup of orange juice.

        1-1/2 tablespoons olive oil
        1 medium-size onion, cut in half lengthwise,
           thinly sliced lengthwise (5 oz.)
        1 small garlic clove, pressed *or* minced
        1 (16-oz.) can whole peeled tomatoes
        1 (14-oz.) can artichoke hearts packed in water,
           drained, quartered
        1 bay leaf
        1/2 teaspoon dried basil
        8 oz. linguini, fettucini *or* spaghetti

In a medium-size skillet heat oil over medium heat. Add onion and garlic; cook until onion is soft but not browned. Pour tomatoes and their liquid into pan; coarsely cut up tomatoes. Add artichoke hearts, bay leaf and basil. Bring to a boil over high heat; reduce heat. Cover; simmer 10 minutes. Uncover; simmer 5 minutes or until sauce thickens slightly. Remove bay leaf. In a large kettle of boiling water, cook linguini 8 to 10 minutes or until tender but firm to the bite; drain. Place in a serving bowl. Add sauce. Toss until pasta is well coated with sauce. Makes 4 (1-1/4 cup) servings.

PER SERVING: 1-1/4 cups

CALORIES	CARBOHYDRATES	PROTEIN	FAT	CHOLESTEROL
256	47 gm	8 gm	6 gm	0 mg

Eggplant Lasagne

An hour of weekend cooking will do wonders for a hurry-up weekday meal. It allows you to take time to work out, then sit down for a nourishing meal. Serve this lasagne with a crisp green salad and garlic bread.

> 1 large eggplant, unpeeled, cut crosswise in
>   1/4-inch-thick slices (1-1/4 lbs.)
> 1 pkg. whole-wheat *or* regular lasagne noodles (8 oz.)
> 4 cups Marinara Sauce (page 138) *or* purchased
>   marinara sauce
> 1-1/2 cups low-fat cottage cheese
> 1-1/2 cups shredded part-skim mozzarella cheese (6 oz.)
> 3 tablespoons grated Parmesan cheese

Preheat oven to 400F (205C). Grease a large baking sheet with vegetable nonstick cooking spray. Place eggplant slices in a single layer on prepared baking sheet. Bake eggplant in preheated oven 18 minutes or until tender. Remove from oven; let cool 10 minutes. In a large kettle of boiling water, cook lasagne 10 minutes or until tender but firm to the bite. Drain, rinse with cold water and drain again. Grease a 13″ x 9″ baking pan with vegetable nonstick cooking spray; spread a thin layer of marinara sauce over the bottom. Arrange 1/3 of noodles over sauce. Cover with 1/2 the eggplant; top with 1/2 of the cottage cheese. Cover cottage cheese with 1/3 of sauce. Sprinkle 1/3 of the mozzarella cheese evenly over sauce. Make another layer using 1/3 of noodles, remaining eggplant, remaining cottage cheese, 1/3 of sauce, and 1/3 of mozzarella. Complete the final layer with the remaining noodles, sauce and mozzarella. Sprinkle Parmesan cheese over top. If made ahead, cover and refrigerate up to 2 days. Bake, covered, in a 350F (175C) oven 50 minutes (60 minutes if refrigerated) or until hot and bubbly. Cut in squares to serve. Makes 8 servings.

PER SERVING: 1/8 of total recipe

CALORIES	CARBOHYDRATES	PROTEIN	FAT	CHOLESTEROL
198	24 gm	12 gm	6 gm	13 mg

Creole Rice

Whoever said that carbohydrates have to be boring? This dish is redolent with allspice and bay and especially tasty with the fruitiness of plump raisins. For a memorable meal, serve it alongside Chicken Breasts with Hot Marmalade Sauce, page 99, and steamed broccoli.

1 tablespoon vegetable oil
1/2 cup chopped onion
1 garlic clove, pressed *or* minced
1/2 cup chopped green bell pepper
1 (16-oz.) can whole peeled tomatoes
1/2 cup raisins
1/2 teaspoon paprika
1/4 teaspoon ground allspice
1/2 bay leaf
4 drops hot pepper sauce
3 cups cooked long-grain brown *or* long-grain
    white rice (1 cup uncooked)
Salt and pepper to taste

In a large skillet heat oil over medium heat. Add onion, garlic and bell pepper; cook until onion is soft but not browned. Pour tomatoes and their liquid into skillet; coarsely cut up tomatoes. Add raisins, paprika, allspice, bay leaf and hot pepper sauce; bring to a boil over high heat. Reduce heat; simmer, uncovered, 10 minutes or until sauce is thick and chunky. Discard bay leaf. Add rice; stir to completely coat kernels with sauce. Cook 5 minutes or until rice is hot and almost all liquid is absorbed. Season with salt and pepper. Makes 6 servings.

PER SERVING: 1/6 of total recipe				
CALORIES	CARBOHYDRATES	PROTEIN	FAT	CHOLESTEROL
181	36 gm	3 gm	3 gm	0 mg

Zucchini-Rice Quiche

Hearty and wholesome, this meatless quiche can be whipped up with ease. The rice crust is a good source of complex carbohydrates, the kind of food that fills you up without rounding you out. To double the fiber, use brown rice in place of white.

2 tablespoons wheat germ
3 cups cold cooked long-grain white rice (1 cup uncooked)
2 tablespoons margarine
3 medium-size zucchini, cut in 1/8-inch-thick
    slices (1 lb. *total*)
1 cup shredded farmer cheese (4 oz.)
1 cup part-skim ricotta cheese (8 oz.)
3 eggs
1/2 cup skim milk
1/2 teaspoon salt
White pepper to taste
1/4 teaspoon garlic powder
1/2 teaspoon dried oregano
1/2 teaspoon dried basil

Grease a 10-inch pie pan with vegetable nonstick cooking spray. Sprinkle wheat germ evenly over bottom and sides of pie pan. Press cooked, cooled rice over bottom of pan and 2/3 of the way up sides to form a shell. Preheat oven to 350F (175C). In a medium-size skillet melt margarine over medium-high heat. Add zucchini. Cook, uncovered, stirring occasionally, until zucchini is crisp-tender. Arrange 1/2 of zucchini over bottom of rice crust. Sprinkle farmer cheese evenly over zucchini. In a large bowl, combine ricotta cheese, eggs, milk, salt, white pepper, garlic powder, oregano and basil; stir until smooth. Pour into pie pan. Arrange remaining zucchini on top; filling should just barely cover edges of rice crust. Bake in preheated oven 35 to 40 minutes or until a knife inserted in center comes out clean. Cool on a wire rack 10 minutes before serving. Makes 6 servings.

PER SERVING: 1/6 of total recipe				
CALORIES	CARBOHYDRATES	PROTEIN	FAT	CHOLESTEROL
296	29 gm	15 gm	13 gm	161 mg

Minted Spinach & Rice

Lemon and mint give a refreshing lift to this side dish that makes a fabulous accompaniment to Grilled Persian Lamb, page 91. High in complex carbohydrates, this recipe is loaded with nutrients that are important for the active person. One serving supplies over 100% of the US RDA for vitamins A and C, and provides almost 25% of the US RDA for iron. The high vitamin C content enables more of the iron to be absorbed.

3/4 lb. spinach, washed, stems removed,
   coarsely chopped
1/4 cup chopped parsley
1 tablespoon chopped fresh mint *or* 1 teaspoon dried mint,
   crumbled
1/4 teaspoon ground nutmeg
1 tablespoon olive oil
1 medium-size onion, chopped (5 oz.)
1 garlic clove, pressed *or* minced
1/2 cup uncooked long-grain white rice
1/2 cup water
1/2 cup canned tomato sauce
Salt and pepper to taste
1 lemon, cut in wedges

In a large bowl, combine spinach, parsley, mint and nutmeg; set aside. In a 3-quart saucepan heat oil over medium heat. Add onion and garlic; cook until onion is soft but not browned. Stir in rice; cook, stirring for 2 minutes. Add water and tomato sauce; bring to a boil over high heat. Reduce heat; cover and simmer 20 minutes or until rice is tender and almost all liquid is absorbed. Add spinach mixture; thoroughly stir into rice. Cover; cook 5 minutes or until spinach is wilted. Season with salt and pepper. Serve with lemon wedges to squeeze over each serving. Makes 4 servings.

PER SERVING: 2/3 cup				
CALORIES	CARBOHYDRATES	PROTEIN	FAT	CHOLESTEROL
166	29 gm	5 gm	4 gm	0 mg

Chiles Rellenos

You can do some pretty fancy things with chiles without putting forth much effort. Here is one tasty example that you can serve as a meatless entree or as a side-dish to accompany grilled chicken or fish.

> 1 cup cooked long-grain white rice (1/3 cup uncooked rice)
> 1 cup cooked corn *or* 1 (8-oz.) can whole-kernel corn, drained
> 2 green onions, thinly sliced, including tops
> 1/2 cup low-fat cottage cheese
> 1 cup shredded farmer cheese (4 oz.)
> Pepper to taste
> 2 (7-oz. *each*) cans whole green chiles
> 3/4 cup Ten-Minute Salsa (page 56) *or* purchased salsa

In a medium-size bowl, combine rice, corn, green onions, cottage cheese, farmer cheese and pepper. Grease a 13" x 9" baking pan with vegetable nonstick cooking spray. Preheat oven to 350F (175C). Slice each chile carefully down one side; remove seeds and pith. Place 1/4 cup of filling in each chili; gently reform chili to make a boat shape. Arrange filled chiles, side-by-side in baking dish; cover with aluminum foil. Bake in preheated oven 30 minutes or until chiles are hot and cheese is melted. Use a wide spatula to transfer chiles to each serving plate. Spoon 2 tablespoon salsa over each serving. Makes 6 servings of 2 chiles each.

PER SERVING: 2 stuffed chiles

CALORIES	CARBOHYDRATES	PROTEIN	FAT	CHOLESTEROL
141	19 gm	7 gm	5 gm	9 mg

Working With Chiles:
Chiles contain volatile oils which may make your skin burn and your eyes smart. Avoid touching your face while working with chiles. After handling chiles wash your hands well with soap and water.

Asparagus Rice with Creamy Seafood Sauce

In typical Chinese fashion, this high-carbohydrate dish uses a little bit of protein for garnish. The result is an entree that is as lovely to see as it is to taste. Each serving is a good source of iron and contains less fat than a tablespoon of blue cheese salad dressing.

1/3 lb. scallops *or* surimi-style (imitation) crabmeat
1-1/2 cups regular-strength chicken broth
1-1/2 tablespoons cornstarch
1-1/2 lbs. asparagus
1 tablespoon vegetable oil
1/2 teaspoon minced fresh gingerroot
2 teaspoons dry sherry
1 egg, lightly beaten
4 cups hot cooked long-grain white rice (1-1/3 cups uncooked)
1 lemon, cut in wedges

If using large sea scallops, cut in thirds; leave bay scallops whole. If using crabmeat, coarsely flake. Set seafood aside. In a small bowl, blend chicken broth and cornstarch until smooth. Snap off and discard tough asparagus ends. Place asparagus in a wide skillet with 1 inch of boiling water. Simmer 4 to 5 minutes or until not quite crisp-tender; turn off heat. In a large skillet heat oil over medium heat. Add ginger; stir-fry 10 seconds. Add scallops and sherry; stir-fry 2 minutes or until scallops become opaque. (If using crab, add with sherry; stir-fry 1 minute.) Stir chicken broth-cornstarch mixture once to recombine; add to skillet. Cook, stirring, until sauce comes to a gentle boil and slightly thickens. Remove skillet from heat. Add egg to sauce; stir until it forms long threads. To serve, spoon 1 cup of rice onto each of 4 plates. Drain asparagus; evenly divide among plates and arrange over rice. Spoon seafood sauce over asparagus. Serve with lemon wedges to squeeze over each serving. Makes 4 servings.

PER SERVING: 1/4 of total recipe				
CALORIES	CARBOHYDRATES	PROTEIN	FAT	CHOLESTEROL
323	51 gm	17 gm	6 gm	86 mg

Wheat Berries with Sweet Peppers & Tofu

Wheat berries (whole wheat kernels) are not something you think about having for dinner on your way home from work. Advance planning is necessary as they take two hours to cook. High in fiber, this grain makes a nice change from rice and is worth cooking ahead and freezing. One cup uncooked wheat berries will yield about three cups cooked grain. If you can't find wheat berries substitute 4 cups cooked brown rice.

    1-1/3 cups uncooked whole wheat berries
    5 cups water
    1-1/2 tablespoons vegetable oil
    1 medium-size onion, chopped (5 oz.)
    1 garlic clove, pressed *or* minced
    2 medium-size red bell peppers, seeded, cored,
        diced (12 oz. *total*)
    1/2 teaspoon ground cumin
    1/2 teaspoon dried oregano
    12 oz. regular *or* firm tofu, rinsed drained,
        cut in 1/2-inch cakes
    2 tablespoons red wine vinegar
    1 teaspoon Worcestershire sauce
    12 oz. spinach, washed, stems removed,
        coarsely chopped
    Salt and pepper to taste

In a 3-quart saucepan combine wheat berries and water. Bring to a boil over high heat; cover. Reduce heat; simmer 2 hours or until berries are tender to bite; drain well. In a large nonstick skillet heat oil over medium heat. Add onion, garlic and bell peppers. Cook until onion is soft but not browned. Stir in cumin and oregano; cook 30 seconds. Add tofu, wine vinegar and Worcestershire. Cook 3 minutes or until tofu is lightly browned. Add cooked wheat berries and spinach. Stir gently but thoroughly until ingredients are evenly mixed. Cover skillet; cook 5 minutes or until wheat berries are hot and spinach is wilted. Add salt and pepper to taste. Makes 6 servings.

PER SERVING: 1/6 of total recipe				
CALORIES	CARBOHYDRATES	PROTEIN	FAT	CHOLESTEROL
245	39 gm	10 gm	7 gm	0 mg

Marinara Sauce

The easiest way to change pasta from fattening fare to fitness food is to cut out the white sauce made from cream, butter and cheese, and substitute this thick garden-fresh tomato sauce that is chock-full of nutrients. Use the sauce alone or add sliced mushrooms or a bit of browned lean ground beef for a variation in flavor.

2 tablespoons olive oil
1 large onion, chopped (7 oz.)
1 medium-size carrot, chopped (4 oz.)
1 celery stalk, chopped
4 garlic cloves, pressed *or* minced
2 tablespoons tomato paste
2 (28-oz. *each*) cans whole peeled tomatoes
1/2 cup dry red wine
1 bay leaf
1 teaspoon dried basil
1 teaspoon dried oregano
1/4 teaspoon ground cloves
Salt and pepper to taste

In a 3-quart saucepan heat oil over medium heat. Add onion, carrot, celery and garlic; cook until onion is soft but not browned. Stir in tomato paste. Add tomatoes and their liquid; coarsely cut up tomatoes. Add wine, bay leaf, basil, oregano and cloves. Bring to a boil over high heat; reduce heat. Simmer, uncovered, 1 hour. Remove bay leaf. In a blender, process sauce, a portion at a time, to make a smooth puree. Measure sauce; if less than 7 cups, add water to make 7 cups. If more than 7 cups, return to kettle; simmer until reduced to 7 cups. Add salt and pepper to taste; let cool. Cover and refrigerate up to 1 week, or pour into 1 cup containers and freeze. Makes 7 cups.

PER SERVING: 1 cup

CALORIES	CARBOHYDRATES	PROTEIN	FAT	CHOLESTEROL
98	11 gm	2 gm	4 gm	0 mg

Quick Tomato Sauce

This all-purpose sauce is a great source of vitamins A and C, and surprisingly, a good source of iron, especially if you cook in a cast-iron skillet. It's similar in thickness to canned tomato sauce, but more flavorful.

1 tablespoon olive oil
1 medium-size onion, finely chopped (5 oz.)
1 garlic clove, pressed *or* minced
1 (28-oz.) can whole peeled tomatoes
3 tablespoons tomato paste
1 (14-1/2-oz.) can regular-strength chicken broth *or*
    1-3/4 cups homemade chicken broth
1/2 teaspoon dried basil
1/2 teaspoon dried oregano
Salt and pepper to taste

In a large skillet heat oil over medium heat. Add onion and garlic; cook until onion is soft but not browned. Combine tomatoes and their liquid and tomato paste in a blender or food processor. Process until pureed. Pour into skillet; add chicken broth, basil and oregano. Bring to a boil over high heat; reduce heat. Simmer, uncovered, 30 minutes or until sauce is the consistency of canned tomato sauce. Add salt and pepper to taste; let cool. Cover and refrigerate up to 1 week, or pour into 1 cup containers and freeze. Makes 4 cups.

PER SERVING: 1 cup

CALORIES	CARBOHYDRATES	PROTEIN	FAT	CHOLESTEROL
124	19 gm	5 gm	4 gm	6 mg

Zorba Pocket Sandwiches

Here is a Middle Eastern sandwich for which Zorba the Greek would dance. Even though it is meatless, this whole-meal sandwich is high in protein, low in fat, and contains generous amounts of iron and vitamin C. Make it easy on yourself; serve everything at the table and let each person build his sandwich.

1 (15-oz.) can garbanzo beans, drained
1/4 cup tahini (sesame seed paste)
3 tablespoons lemon juice
1 garlic clove, pressed *or* minced
1/2 teaspoon ground coriander
1/2 teaspoon ground cumin
1/2 teaspoon salt
1/4 teaspoon chili powder
1/4 cup water
6 (6-inch) whole-wheat *or* regular pocket breads,
   cut in half crosswise

Garnishes:
1-1/2 cups alfalfa sprouts *or* 1-1/2 cups shredded
   iceberg lettuce
3 medium-size tomatoes, diced (15 oz. *total*)
3 green onions, thinly sliced, including tops
12 radishes, thinly sliced
1-1/2 cups plain low-fat yogurt

In a food processor or blender, combine garbanzo beans, tahini, lemon juice, garlic, coriander, cumin, salt, chili powder and water. Process until mixture is smooth. Spoon into a small serving bowl. Place bread halves in a basket. Place alfalfa sprouts, tomatoes, green onions, radishes and yogurt in individual bowls. Set all ingredients on the table. Each person assembles the sandwich in the following manner: Spread about 2 tablespoons garbanzo puree in each bread pocket; top with sprouts, tomato, green onion and a few radish slices. Spoon a dollop of yogurt over top of each pocket sandwich. Makes 6 servings of 2 pocket sandwiches each.

PER SERVING: 2 pocket sandwiches

CALORIES	CARBOHYDRATES	PROTEIN	FAT	CHOLESTEROL
318	50 gm	16 gm	6 gm	1 mg

VEGETABLES

The vegetable world offers such vast choices of seasonal flavors, colors, and textures you can rely on it day-after-day to give a fresh twist to meal planning. Vegetables provide dietary fiber, and are a powerhouse of vitamins and minerals as well. Take advantage of vegetables in season to come up with your own simple recipes.

The vegetables in this chapter are easy and quick to prepare. Broccoli-Stuffed Onions, page 146, can serve as a centerpiece for a colorful fall buffet, as well as supply part of your daily requirements for vitamin C. Basil Squash, page 149, cooks in 2 minutes and tastes like it was just picked from the garden. Another time, top these bright yellow and green shreds of summer squash with marinara sauce for an easy vegetable "pasta." Asparagus Milanese, page 142, makes a fine salute to spring.

STEAMED, MICROWAVED & STIR-FRIED VEGETABLES

When you want to serve a simple unadorned vegetable accompaniment, steaming and microwaving are two popular ways to prepare vegetables. Both cooking methods seal in vitamins and minerals and are an easy and quick way to cook. Follow directions in a microwave cookbook for method and times. For maximum speed and flavor that doesn't need a boost of a sauce, try stir-frying. For 1 pound (4 servings) of cut-up vegetables, heat 1 tablespoon of vegetable oil in a wok or skillet. Add vegetables to the hot wok and toss for 1 minute. Drizzle 1 tablespoon of water down the wok sides, cover, and cook until you hear the wok sizzle. If vegetables are not yet crisp-tender, add another tablespoon of water and repeat. Just before the vegetables are ready to serve, sprinkle them with seasonings. Try rosemary with stir-fried broccoli flowerets and sliced mushrooms; dill with cauliflower flowerets and sliced carrots; or basil with zucchini and red bell pepper strips. Chinese cooks season the wok by cooking a pinch of minced garlic and fresh gingerroot in the hot oil before adding the vegetables. You may chose to do this. If you like Oriental seasonings, go easy on the soy sauce. One tablespoon contains 1029 mg of sodium, about the same amount of sodium as is in 1/2 teaspoon of salt.

Stuffed Artichokes, Italian Style

You won't miss a fat-laden mayonnaise or Hollandaise sauce with these artichokes. The savory stuffing tucked into the leaves provides plenty of flavor. Serve them warm or at room temperature.

> 4 medium-size artichokes (6 oz. *each*)
> 1/2 lemon
> 1/2 cup seasoned Italian-style dry bread crumbs
> 2 tablespoons grated Parmesan cheese
> 1 green onion, finely chopped, including top
> 1/8 teaspoon pepper
> 2 tablespoons olive oil
> 2 tablespoons distilled white vinegar
> 1/4 teaspoon salt
> 4 cherry tomatoes

Cut off artichoke stems so they stand level. Remove and discard small coarse outer leaves. Cut off top one-third of each artichoke. Using scissors, cut off thorny tips of remaining leaves. Rinse well. Rub cut surfaces with lemon half. Separate leaves of each artichoke enough to insert a spoon; set aside. In a bowl, combine bread crumbs, Parmesan cheese, green onion and pepper. Allowing 2-1/2 tablespoons of stuffing for each artichoke, tuck stuffing firmly down between leaves. Drizzle 1-1/2 teaspoons olive oil over stuffing in each artichoke. Stand artichokes, stuffing side-up, in a kettle, with a lid, that is just large enough to hold artichokes snugly in place. Sprinkle vinegar and salt between artichokes. Pour in water to a depth of 1 inch; cover. Bring to a boil over high heat; reduce heat. Simmer 25 to 30 minutes or until artichokes are tender when pierced with a fork at the stem ends. Lift out artichokes with a slotted spoon; drain on paper towels. Let stand 30 minutes before serving. If made ahead, cool, cover and refrigerate; bring to room temperature before serving. Garnish the top of each artichoke with a cherry tomato. Makes 4 servings.

PER SERVING: 1 artichoke				
CALORIES	CARBOHYDRATES	PROTEIN	FAT	CHOLESTEROL
185	23 gm	6 gm	8 gm	2 mg

Asparagus Milanese

With fresh asparagus, the simplest preparation is often the best way to enjoy the flavor and utilize its vitamin C.

> 1-1/3 lbs. asparagus
> 1-1/2 teaspoons lemon juice
> 1-1/2 teaspoons olive oil
> Salt and pepper to taste
> 1 tablespoon grated Parmesan cheese

Snap off and discard tough asparagus ends. Place asparagus in a wide skillet with 1 inch of boiling water; cover. Simmer 6 to 8 minutes or until spears are tender when pierced; drain. Place on heated serving platter; drizzle with lemon juice and olive oil. Sprinkle with salt and pepper to taste, then sprinkle with Parmesan cheese. Serve hot. Makes 4 servings.

PER SERVING: 1/4 of total recipe				
CALORIES	CARBOHYDRATES	PROTEIN	FAT	CHOLESTEROL
62	6 gm	5 gm	2 gm	0 mg

Green Beans in Wine

Vitamin A, potassium, and fiber are the benefits you reap from eating fresh green beans.

2 teaspoons olive oil
1 garlic clove, pressed *or* minced
1 medium-size tomato, peeled, seeded, chopped (5 oz.) *or*
   1/2 cup canned tomatoes and their liquid
1 lb. green beans, ends removed, cut in 2-inch lengths
1 tablespoon chopped parsley
1 teaspoon dried basil
1/3 cup dry red wine
Salt and pepper to taste

In a saucepan heat oil over medium heat. Add garlic; cook for 30 seconds. Add tomato, green beans, parsley and basil; mix well. Cook, uncovered, for 3 minutes. Add wine. Bring to a boil over high heat; cover and reduce heat. Simmer 8 to 10 minutes or until beans are crisp-tender. Add salt and pepper to taste. Makes 4 servings.

PER SERVING: 1/4 of total recipe

CALORIES	CARBOHYDRATES	PROTEIN	FAT	CHOLESTEROL
71	8 gm	2 gm	3 gm	0 mg

Pickled Beets

Try this cool vegetable side-dish on a hot summer day. It's a bargain in calories and a fat-free way to add spice to a meal of barbecued chicken.

1-1/2 lbs. beets *or* 1 (16-oz.) can sliced beets, drained
2 tablespoons distilled white vinegar
2 tablespoons water
1 tablespoon sugar
1/2 teaspoon caraway seeds
1 teaspoon prepared horseradish
Salt to taste
4 watercress sprigs

Scrub fresh beets well. Leave on roots and 2 inches of stem. Do not peel. Place beets in a saucepan; add water to cover. Bring to a boil over high heat; reduce heat. Simmer, covered, 30 to 40 minutes or until beets are tender when pierced; drain. Let cool; trim off roots and stems; slip off skins. Cut beets crosswise in 1/8-inch-thick slices. In a plastic bag, mix vinegar, the 2 tablespoons water, sugar, caraway seeds, horseradish and salt to taste. Add beet slices to bag; seal. Turn bag over to distribute marinade. Refrigerate for at least 2 hours or as long as overnight; turn bag occasionally to distribute marinade. To serve, lift beets from marinade with a slotted spoon. Place on a serving plate; garnish with watercress. Makes 4 (1/2-cup) servings.

PER SERVING: 1/2 cup

CALORIES	CARBOHYDRATES	PROTEIN	FAT	CHOLESTEROL
43	10 gm	1 gm	0 gm	0 mg

Red Cabbage & Apples

Recent nutritional surveys show that cruciferous vegetables—the various forms of cabbage, broccoli, Brussels sprouts, cauliflower, kale, kohlrabi and turnip greens, are an important part of a healthy eating plan. Cabbage is a cruciferous vegetable rich in minerals, vitamins A and C and an excellent source of dietary fiber. Teamed with apples, this sweet-sour vegetable makes a good accompaniment to roast turkey or steamed turkey sausages.

> 1 tablespoon margarine
> 4 cups cored, finely shredded red cabbage (*about* 1 lb.)
> 2 medium-size apples, Granny Smith *or* Golden Delicious,
>   peeled, cored, chopped (12 oz. *total*)
> 2 tablespoons water
> 1/4 cup red wine vinegar
> 2 tablespoons honey
> 1/4 teaspoon ground nutmeg
> Salt and pepper to taste

In a skillet melt margarine over medium heat. Add cabbage and apples; cook for 4 minutes or until cabbage begins to wilt. Add water, wine vinegar and honey. Cover; simmer 20 minutes or until cabbage is crisp-tender. Uncover; increase heat to high. Cook, shaking pan, until most of liquid has evaporated. Add nutmeg and salt and pepper to taste. Makes 4 servings.

PER SERVING: 1/4 of total recipe

CALORIES	CARBOHYDRATES	PROTEIN	FAT	CHOLESTEROL
143	29 gm	2 gm	4 gm	0 mg

Sherried Carrots

Here's a quick way to make the common carrot special. One serving supplies 130% of the US RDA for vitamin A.

> 1 lb. carrots, peeled, cut in 1/4-inch-thick slices
> Water
> 1 tablespoon margarine
> 1-1/2 tablespoons dry sherry
> 2 green onion tops, thinly sliced
> Salt and pepper to taste

In a medium-size saucepan, cook carrots, covered, in 1/2-inch simmering water 8 to 10 minutes or until tender; drain. Add margarine, sherry, green onion tops and salt and pepper to taste. Cook over medium heat, shaking pan, until most of liquid evaporates and carrots are lightly browned on all sides. Makes 4 servings.

PER SERVING: 1/4 of total recipe

CALORIES	CARBOHYDRATES	PROTEIN	FAT	CHOLESTEROL
82	12 gm	1 gm	3 gm	0 mg

Cauliflower with Capers

Served hot, this tastes fabulous with grilled fish or meat. To serve at room temperature, offer it with Marinated Mushrooms, page 59, for an easy antipasto. One serving supplies 68% of the vitamin C you need each day.

> 1 medium-size head cauliflower, trimmed, broken into
>   flowerets (1-1/4 lbs.)
> 1 tablespoon olive oil
> 1 garlic clove, pressed *or* minced
> 2 tablespoons capers, rinsed, drained, chopped
> 3 tablespoons white wine vinegar
> 2 tablespoons chopped parsley
> Salt and pepper to taste

Place cauliflower in a wide skillet with 1/2 inch of boiling water; cover. Simmer 5 to 8 minutes or until tender when pierced; drain well and set aside. In a large skillet heat oil over medium heat. Add garlic; cook for 1 minute. Add capers, wine vinegar and parsley; cook for 2 minutes. Add cauliflower. Shake pan and toss cauliflower until heated through and evenly coated with seasonings. Add salt and pepper to taste. Serve hot, or cool and serve at room temperature. Makes 6 servings.

PER SERVING: 1/6 of total recipe

CALORIES	CARBOHYDRATES	PROTEIN	FAT	CHOLESTEROL
50	6 gm	2 gm	2 gm	0 mg

Grilled Eggplant

Barbecuing allows you to cook eggplant without any oil. To have a vegetable that stays juicy, you must use the long slender Oriental variety. Serve this with grilled fish.

> 1 tablespoon soy sauce
> 1/4 cup regular-strength chicken broth
> 1 teaspoon grated fresh gingerroot
> Red (cayenne) pepper to taste
> 4 Oriental eggplant (1 lb. *total*)

In a small bowl, combine soy, chicken broth, ginger and red pepper to taste; divide equally among 4 small dipping sauce bowls. Place whole eggplant on a lightly greased grill 4 to 6 inches above a solid bed of low-glowing coals. Cook, turning often, 10 to 15 minutes or until eggplant is soft when pierced. Provide each diner with a bowl of dipping sauce. Use the mixture as a dip for each bite-full of eggplant. Makes 4 servings.

PER SERVING: 1/4 of total recipe

CALORIES	CARBOHYDRATES	PROTEIN	FAT	CHOLESTEROL
27	6 gm	1 gm	0 gm	0 mg

Caramelized Onion & Spinach

As a change from creamed spinach, try this spinach with a mild sweet-sour flavor. It is a good source of vitamins A and C and supplies 15% of the US RDA for iron. Don't rush the onion, it needs to cook slowly for 30 minutes to become mellow and sweet.

1 tablespoon vegetable oil
1 large onion, cut in half lengthwise, thinly sliced (7 oz.)
1/2 teaspoon sugar
1 bunch spinach, washed, stems removed,
   lightly drained (12 oz.)
1 tablespoon lemon juice
Salt and pepper to taste

In a large skillet heat oil over medium heat. Add onion; cook for 10 minutes. Reduce heat to medium-low; cook, stirring occasionally, for 15 minutes or until onion is very soft and golden brown. Stir in sugar; cook for 5 minutes or until onion is caramelized and flecked with dark brown bits. Add spinach; cover. Cook 2 minutes. Turn spinach leaves over. Cover; cook 3 minutes longer or until spinach is wilted but still bright green. Uncover; increase heat to high and cook until most of liquid has evaporated. Stir in lemon juice and salt and pepper to taste. Heat through. Makes 4 servings.

PER SERVING: 1/4 of total recipe				
CALORIES	CARBOHYDRATES	PROTEIN	FAT	CHOLESTEROL
74	9 gm	3 gm	4 gm	0 mg

Broccoli-Stuffed Onions

On their own, these stuffed onions make a handsome vegetable dish to serve on a buffet. Or serve them on either end of a platter to accompany a whole roast chicken or game hens. Choose onions which are flatly rounded rather than oval shape, so they will make non-tipable containers. Each stuffed onion supplies almost half the amount of vitamin C you need each day.

4 medium-size onions (5 oz. *each*)
2/3 cup chopped cooked broccoli
2 tablespoons dry bread crumbs
2 teaspoons olive oil
2 teaspoons grated Parmesan cheese
1/4 teaspoon dried rosemary
Salt and pepper to taste

Preheat oven to 350F (175C). Place unpeeled onions in a 9-inch square pan. Bake, un-covered, for 30 to 40 minutes or until onions are tender when pierced. Let cool. Peel onions. Using a curved grapefruit knife, cut out core from center of each onion leaving a 1/2-inch-thick shell. If a hole appears in bottom of onion, cover with a layer of cooked onion. Coarsely chop 2 tablespoons of cooked onion centers; save remaining centers for other uses if desired. In a small bowl, combine chopped onion, broccoli, bread crumbs, olive oil, Parmesan cheese, rosemary and salt and pepper to taste; mix well. Stuff onion shells with broccoli mixture. Wash and dry pan; grease with vegetable nonstick cooking spray. Place onions in pan. Bake, covered, in a 350F (175C) oven for 30 minutes or until filling is hot. Makes 4 servings.

PER SERVING: 1 onion				
CALORIES	CARBOHYDRATES	PROTEIN	FAT	CHOLESTEROL
69	10 gm	3 gm	3 gm	0 mg

Peas with Onions

Tiny cocktail-size onions, called pearl onions, add delicious sweetness to peas and boost the potassium content of this mineral-packed vegetable dish.

1 (10-oz.) pkg. frozen pearl onions
2 teaspoons margarine
2 tablespoons sugar
1/4 cup dry white wine
1 (10-oz.) pkg. frozen green peas
1/2 cup regular-strength chicken broth
White pepper to taste

In a 2-quart saucepan, combine onions, margarine, sugar and wine. Cook, uncovered, over medium heat for 5 minutes or until onions are thawed and just begin to soften. Add peas and chicken stock. Cover; simmer for 3 minutes or until peas are tender. Add pepper to taste. Makes 6 servings.

PER SERVING: 1/6 of total recipe				
CALORIES	CARBOHYDRATES	PROTEIN	FAT	CHOLESTEROL
87	14 gm	3 gm	2 gm	1 mg

Oven French Fries

Here is an easy way to satisfy your craving for French fries and still have food that is good for you. The same serving of fries from a fast food restaurant would have 275 calories and 14 grams of fat. From commercially prepared frozen oven fries the same amount would have 245 calories and 13 grams fat.

> **3 medium-size russet potatoes (1-1/4 lbs. *total*)**
> **1 tablespoon vegetable oil**
> **1 tablespoon Dijon-style mustard**
> **1 tablespoon water**
> **Salt and pepper to taste**

Preheat oven to 425F (220C). Scrub unpeeled potatoes well; dry. Cut in half lengthwise; cut each half into finger-width wedges. In a medium-size bowl, combine oil, mustard, and water; whisk until blended. Add half of potato wedges to bowl; turn to coat all sides. Lift wedges from bowl, allowing excess liquid to drip back into bowl. Arrange in a single layer in a 15" x 10" rimmed baking pan. Repeat with remaining potato wedges. Sprinkle with salt and pepper to taste. Bake, uncovered, in preheated oven for 20 minutes. Turn wedges over. Bake for 20 more minutes or until potatoes are golden brown. Makes 4 servings.

PER SERVING: 1/4 of total recipe

CALORIES	CARBOHYDRATES	PROTEIN	FAT	CHOLESTEROL
142	25 gm	3 gm	4 gm	0 mg

Skillet Potatoes

Potatoes are good for you—possibly in more ways than you have ever imagined. They are a good source of vitamin C and they contain a balance of essential amino acids, the building blocks of protein.

> **1 tablespoon vegetable oil**
> **1 medium-size onion, cut in half, thinly sliced (5 oz.)**
> **1 small garlic clove, pressed *or* minced**
> **1 lb. russet potatoes, peeled, cut in 1/8-inch-thick slices**
> **1/2 teaspoon dried oregano**
> **1 cup regular-strength chicken broth**
> **Salt to taste**

In a wide skillet heat oil over medium heat. Add onion and garlic; cook until onion is soft but not browned. Add potatoes and oregano; stir to mix well. Pour chicken broth over potatoes. Liquid should just barely cover top of potatoes; if not, add water to make up the difference. Bring to a simmer over high heat; reduce heat. Simmer, uncovered, for 30 minutes or until most of liquid has evaporated and potatoes are tender when pierced. Add salt to taste. Makes 4 servings.

PER SERVING: 1/4 of total recipe

CALORIES	CARBOHYDRATES	PROTEIN	FAT	CHOLESTEROL
129	21 gm	4 gm	4 gm	3 mg

Basil Squash

Cook this vegetable dish just until the squash becomes limp. If cooked a minute longer the squash shreds become watery. This summer vegetable dish makes a colorful accompaniment to barbecued chicken or meat.

1/2 lb. zucchini
1/2 lb. crookneck squash
2 teaspoons vegetable oil
1 garlic clove, pressed *or* minced
2 tablespoons regular-strength chicken broth
1 tablespoon chopped fresh basil *or* 1 teaspoon dried basil
Salt and pepper to taste

Using the shredding blade of a food processor or the small holes on a hand grater, shred zucchini and crookneck squash into spaghetti-like strands. In a large skillet heat oil over high heat. Add garlic; cook 5 seconds. Add squash and chicken broth. Cook for 2 minutes or until squash becomes limp. Stir in basil and salt and pepper to taste. Makes 4 servings.

PER SERVING: 1/4 of total recipe

CALORIES	CARBOHYDRATES	PROTEIN	FAT	CHOLESTEROL
42	5 gm	1 gm	2 gm	0 mg

Corn-Chili Stuffed Tomatoes

Tomatoes and corn are high-fiber vegetables. One stuffed tomato supplies 89% of the US RDA for vitamin C. Include this colorful dish at your next summer-time buffet.

4 large ripe, firm tomatoes (6 oz. *each*)
1 cup cooked corn kernels *or* 1 (8-oz.) can whole kernel corn,
    drained
2 tablespoons finely chopped onion
2 tablespoons canned diced green chiles
1/4 teaspoon ground cumin
Salt and pepper to taste
1/4 cup soft bread crumbs
1 tablespoon margarine, melted

Preheat oven to 375F (190C). Grease a 9-inch square baking dish with vegetable nonstick cooking spray; set aside. Cut off a thin slice from the top of each tomato; discard. Using a curved grapefruit knife, scoop out pulp and seeds; reserve. Turn tomato shells upside down on paper towels; let drain for 10 minutes. Chop reserved tomato pulp. Place pulp in a sieve; press with a wooden spoon to extract juice; discard juice. In a bowl, combine tomato pulp, corn, onion, chiles, cumin and salt and pepper to taste; mix well. Stuff tomato shells with corn mixture. In a small bowl, combine bread crumbs with margarine. Press 1/4 of crumbs atop each stuffed tomato. Place tomatoes in prepared dish. Bake in preheated oven 20 minutes or until filling is hot and tomatoes are tender but firm to the touch. Serve hot. Makes 4 servings.

PER SERVING: 1 tomato

CALORIES	CARBOHYDRATES	PROTEIN	FAT	CHOLESTEROL
126	22 gm	4 gm	4 gm	0 mg

SALADS

Crisp, ruffled lettuce leaves; crunchy discs of carrot, radish, and zucchini; skinny shreds of purple or green cabbage; luscious sweet, juicy fruit; and the good carbohydrates—potatoes, pasta and grains—provide the inspiration for salads. They are the part of a meal which is packed with nutrients and eating pleasure as well.

Nutritionally, the only rule for salad is to keep it fresh and light. Antipasto Salad, page 159, or Spinach & Apple Salad, opposite, makes a wonderful starter. If you're looking for a side-dish salad, try Ecuadorian Corn Salad, page 153, or Gingered Carrot Salad, page 152. But who says that a salad has to play second fiddle to a meal? When you add protein, such as in the Taco Salad, page 160, or the Chinese Chicken Salad, page 161, you can make it an easy entree.

While most salads are low in calories, the oils in dressings are not. To save calories and fat, be sparing with any dressing containing fat. At home, toss a salad with just enough dressing to lightly coat each bite. In a restaurant, ask for the dressing to be served on the side. If you are at a salad bar, you can control the amount of dressing you use.

Commercial dressings tend to be high in sodium. Become a label reader; many brands list the calories, fat and sodium content on the bottle. Avoid commercially prepared products that contain palm oil, coconut oil or hydrogenated vegetable oil. The following table gives you a breakdown of calories, fat and soduim content of commercialy prepared salad dressings.

COMMERCIALLY PREPARED SALAD DRESSING

	FAT (gm. per TBSP.)	CALORIES (per TBSP.)	SODIUM (per TBSP.)
Thousand Island			
Regular	5.6	59	109
Low-cal.	1.6	24	153
Blue Cheese			
Regular	8.0	77	N.A.
Low-cal.	0.8	11	155
Italian			
Regular	7.1	69	116
Low-cal.	1.5	16	118
Ranch			
Regular	5.7	54	97
Low-cal.	1.8	19	17
French			
Regular	6.9	70	125
Low-cal.	.9	22	128
Creamy Italian	4.5	52	105

Adapted from Pennington, Jean, and Church, Helen. *Food Values of Portions Commonly Used.* 14th Edition, Harper & Row: New York. 1985.

Spinach & Apple Salad

This salad deserves to star as the first course. Follow this piquant opener, if you like, with Hakone Trout, page 119, Sherried Carrots, page 144 and steamed rice.

> Sesame Dressing (recipe below)
> 1 large bunch spinach, washed, stems removed, chilled (12 oz.)
> 1 large celery stalk, thinly sliced
> 2 green onions, thinly sliced, including tops
> 1 large red-skinned apple, quartered, cored, thinly sliced crosswise (10 oz.)
>
> *Sesame Dressing:*
> 1 tablespoon sesame seeds
> 1/4 cup white wine vinegar
> 2 tablespoons sugar
> 2 tablespoons vegetable oil
> 1/4 teaspoon salt
> 1/4 teaspoon paprika
> 2 drops hot pepper sauce

Prepare Sesame Dressing; set aside. Into a large bowl, tear spinach into bite-size pieces. Add celery, green onions and apple. Pour dressing over spinach; toss gently until well mixed. Makes 6 servings.

Sesame Dressing:
Place sesame seeds in a small dry skillet. Toast over low heat, shaking skillet frequently, for 2 minutes or until seeds turn golden and begin to pop. Place seeds in a small bowl. Add wine vinegar, sugar, oil, salt, paprika and hot pepper sauce; stir until sugar dissolves. Makes about 1/2 cup.

PER SERVING: 1/6 of total recipe

CALORIES	CARBOHYDRATES	PROTEIN	FAT	CHOLESTEROL
91	12 gm	2 gm	5 gm	0 mg

Chinese Cabbage Slaw

For a potluck or a picnic, here's a marvelous coleslaw that is high in fiber, vitamin C, potassium and pizazz. Julienne strips of Chinese cabbage give it a mild flavor and exceptional crunch. Save the curly green edges to toss in a green salad another night. For a fancier presentation, line the bowl with the trimmed curly cabbage edges and garnish the salad with small cooked shrimp or crabmeat.

> 1 small head Chinese (also called napa) cabbage
>   (whole head 1-1/4 lbs.)
> 1 medium-size cucumber (8 oz.)
> 1/4 cup sliced water chestnuts
> 2 green onions, thinly sliced, including tops
> 3 tablespoons seasoned rice vinegar *or* 3 tablespoons rice
>   vinegar plus 1-1/2 teaspoons sugar and 1/8 teaspoon salt
> 1 teaspoon sesame oil

Cut cabbage in half lengthwise; remove core. Trim all curly edges from stalks; save if desired. Cut cabbage stalks into matchstick pieces; place in a large bowl with ice water and chill for 20 minutes. Peel cucumber, leaving alternate strips of green for color. Cut in half lengthwise; scoop out and discard seeds. Cut cucumber halves crosswise into 1/8-inch-thick slices. Drain cabbage well. In a bowl, combine cabbage, cucumber, water chestnuts, onions, seasoned rice vinegar and sesame oil. Mix well. Makes 4 (1-cup) servings.

PER SERVING: 1 cup				
CALORIES	CARBOHYDRATES	PROTEIN	FAT	CHOLESTEROL
35	6 gm	1 gm	1 gm	0 mg

Gingered Carrot Salad

This is a sweet and spicy way to take your day's requirement of vitamin A. Serve this refreshing side-dish salad with grilled hamburgers, fish or pork chops.

> 2 tablespoons raisins
> 1 large carrot, grated (1 cup)
> 1 small green onion, with 2 inches of green top, minced
> 2 tablespoons plain low-fat yogurt
> 1/2 teaspoon grated orange peel
> 1 tablespoon orange juice
> 1 teaspoon honey
> 1/2 teaspoon grated fresh gingerroot
> Salt to taste

Place raisins in a medium-size bowl; cover with boiling water. Let stand 15 minutes; drain. Add carrot and green onion; set aside. In a small bowl, combine yogurt, orange peel, orange juice, honey, gingerroot and salt to taste; whisk until evenly blended. Pour dressing over carrot mixture; stir until salad is well moistened. Makes 2 (1/2-cup) servings.

PER SERVING: 1/2 cup				
CALORIES	CARBOHYDRATES	PROTEIN	FAT	CHOLESTEROL
74	18 gm	2 gm	0 gm	0 mg

Ecuadorian Corn Salad

Virtually fat and cholesterol free, this nutrient-dense salad is a good source of iron and vitamins A and C. Serve it at a summer or fall meal when tomatoes are their sweetest.

>   1 small onion (3 oz.)
>   1/2 cup water
>   1/2 cup red wine vinegar
>   1 large tomato (6 oz.)
>   2 cups cooked corn *or* 1 (17-oz.) can whole kernel corn, drained
>   2 tablespoons lime juice
>   2 tablespoons chopped cilantro leaves
>   Salt and red (cayenne) pepper to taste
>   8 butter lettuce leaves

Cut onion in quarters lengthwise; thinly slice each quarter crosswise. In a small bowl, combine onion, water and wine vinegar; marinate for 15 minutes. Drain; discard marinade. Cut tomato in half crosswise; discard seeds. Cut each half in 1/4-inch wedges. In a medium-size bowl, combine marinated onion, tomato, corn, lime juice, cilantro and salt and red pepper to taste; mix lightly. Place 2 lettuce leaves on each of four plates; spoon salad onto lined plates. Makes 4 servings.

PER SERVING: 1/4 of total recipe				
CALORIES	CARBOHYDRATES	PROTEIN	FAT	CHOLESTEROL
91	22 gm	4 gm	1 gm	0 mg

Greek Peasant Salad

Generous amounts of vitamin C, vitamin A and iron are the hidden virtues of this refreshing lemony salad. Serve it with Quick Moussaka, page 82 and crusty bread for an appealing Aegean feast.

>   8 cherry tomatoes, cut in half
>   6 radishes, thinly sliced
>   6 dried cured olives *or* 6 medium-size pitted, whole ripe olives
>   6 flat anchovy fillets, rinsed, drained, coarsely chopped
>   1 small green pepper, seeded, cut in thin rings (4 oz.)
>   1 small red onion, thinly sliced, separated into rings (4 oz.)
>   1 large head romaine, washed, chilled, torn in bite-size pieces
>   1/4 cup olive oil
>   3 tablespoons lemon juice
>   1 garlic clove, pressed *or* minced
>   Salt and freshly ground black pepper to taste

In a large salad bowl, place tomatoes, radishes, olives, anchovies, bell pepper, onion and romaine. If assembled ahead, cover and refrigerate for up to 2 hours. In a small bowl, whisk together oil, lemon juice and garlic. Just before serving, pour dressing over salad; toss gently to mix. Add salt and pepper to taste. Makes 6 servings.

PER SERVING: 1/6 of total recipe				
CALORIES	CARBOHYDRATES	PROTEIN	FAT	CHOLESTEROL
94	5 gm	2 gm	8 gm	2 mg

Mandarin Salad

Sugar-glazed almonds and mandarin oranges give a light touch of sweetness to this first-course salad. If you want a main-dish salad, toss in strips of cooked chicken breast.

> 1/4 cup sliced almonds
> 1/4 cup sugar
> 3 tablespoons vegetable oil
> 2 tablespoons distilled white vinegar
> 1 tablespoon chopped parsley
> 2 drops hot pepper sauce
> 3 cups iceberg lettuce, torn in bite-size pieces (1/2 head)
> 3 cups romaine lettuce, torn in bite-size pieces (1 small head)
> 1 cup sliced celery (2 stalks)
> 2 green onions, thinly sliced, including tops
> 1 (11-oz.) can mandarin oranges, well drained
> Salt and pepper to taste

Combine almonds and 2 tablespoons of the sugar in a small skillet. Place over medium heat. Watch carefully; stir as soon as sugar begins to melt. Continue to stir just until sugar turns a light straw color. Turn candied nuts onto a plate; set aside and let cool. In a small bowl, whisk together oil, the remaining 2 tablespoons sugar, vinegar, parsley and hot pepper sauce. In a large salad bowl, place iceberg lettuce, romaine lettuce, celery, onions and mandarin oranges. Break nuts apart with your fingers to separate; add to salad. Pour dressing over salad; toss gently to mix. Add salt and pepper to taste. Makes 6 servings.

PER SERVING: 1/6 of total recipe				
CALORIES	CARBOHYDRATES	PROTEIN	FAT	CHOLESTEROL
162	17 gm	1 gm	10 gm	0 mg

Garlicky Summer Pasta Salad

Pack this colorful pasta salad in a cooler to share as a finish-line feast after a bike ride or long run. It's a terrific source of vitamin C and complex carbohydrates. To save time, the vegetables can be blanched (parboiled) up to eight hours ahead, covered and refrigerated.

> 2 medium-size leeks (1-1/2-inch diameter)
> 1 cup frozen green peas, thawed
> 1 cup diced zucchini (5 oz.)
> 2 cups broccoli flowerets (1/2 lb.)
> 3 tablespoons olive oil
> 1 tablespoon minced garlic (3 large cloves)
> 1 lb. Italian-style tomatoes *or* regular tomatoes, cored,
>   peeled, coarsely chopped
> 1 tablespoon dried basil
> 8 oz. corkscrew-shaped pasta
> Salt and pepper to taste

Trim and discard ends and tops from leeks leaving about 1-1/2 inches of green leaves. Discard tough outer leaves. Split leeks lengthwise; rinse well. Cut crosswise in 1/4-inch-thick slices. In a 3-quart saucepan, bring 4 inches of water to a rapid boil over high heat. Blanch each type of vegetable by itself. Starting with leeks, drop vegetable into boiling water. Boil, uncovered, about 2 minutes or just until crisp-tender. Lift out with a large slotted spoon and plunge into a large bowl of ice water to stop the cooking action. Then blanch peas and zucchini for about 2 minutes each; plunge into the ice water. Blanch broccoli for 4 minutes and plunge into ice water. When all vegetables are cooled, drain. Spread vegetables out on paper towels and pat dry; set aside. Heat oil in a large skillet over medium heat. Add garlic; cook for 30 seconds. Add tomatoes and basil; cook, stirring for 2 minutes. Remove from heat; let cool. In a large kettle of boiling water, cook pasta 8 to 10 minutes or until tender but firm to the bite. Drain; rinse with cold water; drain again. In a large bowl, combine pasta, tomato-garlic sauce, leeks, peas, zucchini, broccoli, and salt and pepper to taste. Stir gently. Cover and chill for 2 hours or as long as overnight. Makes 8 (1-cup) servings.

PER SERVING: 1 cup				
CALORIES	CARBOHYDRATES	PROTEIN	FAT	CHOLESTEROL
171	25 gm	6 gm	6 gm	0 mg

Tabbuli

No matter where your caravan takes you, this Middle-Eastern salad will hold up well on the hottest of days. It's a nutritious and delicious picnic fare loaded with iron and vitamins A and C. If there are leftovers, spoon tabulli inside of red or green bell pepper halves for a tasty lunch the next day.

> 1 cup bulgur wheat
> 2 cups boiling water
> 2 medium-size tomatoes, seeded, finely diced (10 oz. *total*)
> 5 green onions, finely chopped, including tops
> 1 bunch parsley, chopped (1 cup)
> 1/4 cup chopped fresh mint leaves *or*
>   1-1/2 tablespoons dried mint, crumbled
> 1/2 cup (half 8-oz. can) garbanzo beans, drained
> 1/4 cup olive oil
> 5 tablespoons lemon juice
> 1 teaspoon salt
> 1 teaspoon ground allspice
> 8 romaine lettuce leaves, washed, chilled

In a medium-size bowl, combine bulgur and boiling water. Cover bowl with a plate; let stand for 30 minutes. Drain; add cold water just to cover bulgur. Stir to cool wheat; drain again. Press bulgur between cupped hands to eliminate all water. In a large bowl, combine bulgur, tomatoes, green onions, parsley, mint and garbanzo beans; set aside. In a small bowl, whisk together oil, lemon juice, salt and allspice. Pour dressing over bulgur mixture; stir until well mixed. Serve at once or cover and refrigerate for up to 2 days. To serve, mound tabbuli in a serving bowl; tuck lettuce leaves around inside edges of bowl. To eat, scoop up tabbuli into lettuce leaves. Makes 6 (1-cup) servings.

PER SERVING: 1 cup				
CALORIES	CARBOHYDRATES	PROTEIN	FAT	CHOLESTEROL
226	30 gm	6 gm	10 gm	0 mg

Gazpacho Rice Salad

High in complex carbohydrates and vitamin C, this lightly-dressed salad tastes best freshly made and served at room temperature. When refrigerated, the rice kernels harden slightly because they absorb the dressing. For an easy family meal, serve it with grilled chicken marinated in Texas-Style Barbecue Sauce, page 98.

1 cup uncooked long-grain white rice
1 cup water
1 (8-oz.) can tomato sauce
1 teaspoon salt
1 medium-size cucumber, peeled, seeded, diced (8 oz.)
1/2 *each* medium-size red and green bell pepper, seeded,
   chopped
3 green onions, thinly sliced, including tops
2 tablespoons chopped parsley
3 tablespoons olive oil
3 tablespoons red wine vinegar
1 garlic clove, pressed *or* minced
1/4 teaspoon pepper
1/4 teaspoon dried oregano
1/4 teaspoon dried basil
6 Bibb lettuce *or* other lettuce leaves

In a medium-size saucepan, combine rice, water, tomato sauce, and 1/2 teaspoon of the salt. Cover and bring to a boil over high heat; reduce heat and simmer 20 to 25 minutes or until rice is tender and all liquid is absorbed. Spoon into a large bowl; let cool 30 minutes. Add cucumber, red and green bell pepper, green onions and parsley. In a small bowl, combine oil, wine vinegar, garlic, the remaining 1/2 teaspoon salt, pepper, oregano and basil. Pour dressing over salad and toss gently to mix. Serve at once or cover and let stand at room temperature up to 2 hours. Place a lettuce leaf on each of 6 plates; spoon salad onto center of lettuce lined plates. Or spoon salad into a serving bowl rimmed with lettuce leaves. Make 6 (1-cup) servings.

PER SERVING: 1 cup				
CALORIES	CARBOHYDRATES	PROTEIN	FAT	CHOLESTEROL
192	29 gm	3 gm	7 gm	0 mg

Artichokes Stuffed with Tomato-Eggplant Salad

Here's a great way to cool down after you've exercised in the heat. One artichoke serving has more iron than a 4-ounce hamburger patty. For lunch or a light supper, round out the meal with lavosh crackers, a slice of feta cheese and Creamy Berry Ice, page 178. The components for this salad can be prepared ahead and assembled just before serving.

6 large artichokes (8 oz. *each*)
1/2 lemon
2 tablespoons distilled white vinegar
1 garlic clove, mashed with blade of knife
1 bay leaf
1/4 teaspoon dried oregano

Eggplant-Tomato Salad:
1 medium-size eggplant (1 lb.)
1 garlic clove
1/4 cup olive oil
3 tablespoons white wine vinegar
1 teaspoon dried oregano
Salt and freshly ground black pepper to taste
1 large tomato, diced (6 oz.)
1 tablespoon minced onion
3 tablespoons chopped parsley

Cut off artichoke stems so they stand level. Remove and discard small coarse outer leaves. Cut off top one-third of each artichoke. Using scissors, cut off thorny tips of remaining leaves. Rinse well. Rub cut surfaces with lemon half. Stand artichokes in a 5-quart kettle with a lid. Add vinegar, garlic, bay leaf and oregano. Pour in water to a depth of 2 inches; cover. Bring to a boil over high heat; reduce heat. Simmer 30 to 45 minutes or until artichokes are tender when pierced with a fork at the stem ends; drain. Invert artichokes on paper towels; drain 10 minutes. Remove inside leaves and fuzzy chokes. Use a spoon to scrape out hairy chokes. Cover and refrigerate cooked artichokes until chilled, about 2 hours or for up to 2 days. Prepare Eggplant Tomato Salad. Spoon 1/6 of salad mixture into center of each chilled artichoke. Place 1 filled artichoke on each plate. Drizzle reserved dressing over outer leaves of each artichoke. Makes 6 servings.

Eggplant-Tomato Salad:
Pierce eggplant in several places with a fork. Place on a rimmed baking pan. Bake, uncovered, in a 400F (205C) oven for 50 minutes to 1 hour or until eggplant is fork-tender. Remove from oven; let cool 15 minutes. Peel eggplant; cut flesh into 1/2-inch cubes; set aside. Cut garlic in half. Rub a medium-size bowl with cut sides of garlic; discard garlic. To bowl, add olive oil, wine vinegar, oregano and salt and pepper to taste; stir until blended. Remove half of dressing; reserve. To remaining dressing, add eggplant, tomato, onion, and parsley; mix lightly. Cover and refrigerate eggplant mixture until chilled, about 2 hours or for up to 2 days. If serving the next day, cover reserved dressing and refrigerate; bring to room temperature before using.

PER SERVING: 1/6 of total recipe				
CALORIES	CARBOHYDRATES	PROTEIN	FAT	CHOLESTEROL
234	29 gm	7 gm	10 gm	0 mg

Curried Turkey Salad

A ruffled lettuce leaf and papaya crescents set a perfect stage for this luscious and nutrient-dense salad. Add a basket of Whole Wheat Millet Muffins, page 169, or toasted bagels and you have a sensational summer meal.

       1/4 cup sweetened flaked coconut
       2 cups diced cooked turkey *or* chicken breast
       1 (8-oz.) can pineapple chunks packed in juice, drained
       1/2 cup diced celery
       1/2 cup diced jicama *or* water chestnuts
       1/2 cup plain low-fat yogurt
       1/2 teaspoon curry powder
       1 tablespoon lime juice
       2 tablespoons chopped mango chutney *or* other fruit chutney
       Salt to taste
       8 to 12 Boston lettuce leaves *or* butter lettuce leaves
       1 papaya, peeled, seeded, cut in 8 lengthwise slices

Spread coconut in a shallow rimmed baking pan; toast in a 350F (175C) oven, stirring frequently, for 4 minutes or until lightly browned; set aside. In a large bowl, combine turkey, pineapple, celery and jicama; set aside. In a small bowl, whisk together yogurt, curry powder and 1 teaspoon of the lime juice until smooth. Stir in chutney. Pour dressing over turkey mixture; stir gently to mix. Add salt to taste. Arrange lettuce leaves on 4 plates. Equally mound turkey salad on centers of lettuce-lined plates. Sprinkle the remaining 2 teaspoons lime juice over papaya slices. Arrange 2 papaya slices on either side of turkey mound. Sprinkle 1 tablespoon coconut over each salad. Makes 4 servings.

PER SERVING: 1/4 of total recipe

CALORIES	CARBOHYDRATES	PROTEIN	FAT	CHOLESTEROL
287	30 gm	29 gm	6 gm	72 mg

Tossed Beef Salad with Peaches

When you barbecue or roast beef, cook enough for two meals. This hearty salad is a delicious way to use planned leftovers. The combination of beef, spinach and peaches enhances the amount of iron absorbed by the body.

       1/4 cup vegetable oil
       1/4 cup red wine vinegar
       1 teaspoon prepared horseradish
       1/2 teaspoon Worcestershire sauce
       1/8 teaspoon pepper
       2 drops hot pepper sauce
       3 cups romaine lettuce (1/2 large head)
       3 cups spinach, washed, stems removed,
         well drained (1/2 bunch)
       1-1/2 cups cooked roast beef, cut in julienne strips
       3 small peaches, peeled, pitted, sliced (1-1/2 cups)
       1 small avocado, peeled, pitted, diced
       12 cherry tomatoes, cut in half
       Salt to taste

In a small bowl, whisk together oil, wine vinegar, horseradish, Worcestershire, pepper and hot pepper sauce; set aside. In a large salad bowl, tear lettuce and spinach into bite-size pieces. Add beef, peaches, avocado, and tomatoes. Pour dressing over salad; toss gently to mix. Add salt to taste. Makes 6 servings.

PER SERVING: 1/6 of total recipe				
CALORIES	CARBOHYDRATES	PROTEIN	FAT	CHOLESTEROL
218	11 gm	12 gm	14 gm	27 mg

Antipasto Salad

This easy salad combines the elements of a traditional Italian first course in a delicious whole-meal salad. Served in smaller portions, it makes a great meal teamed up with Pasta With All-Seasons Pesto, page 132.

Antipasto Dressing (recipe below)
1 (6-1/2-oz.) can water-packed tuna, drained, flaked
1 cup broccoli flowerets, blanched, drained, chilled (1 stalk)
1 cup cherry tomatoes, cut in half (1/2 basket)
12 radishes, thinly sliced (1 bunch)
1/4 cup sliced ripe olives
1 medium-size green bell pepper, cut in thin strips (6 oz.)
1 small red onion, thinly sliced (4 oz.)
4 cups romaine lettuce, torn in bite-size pieces (1 small head)
2 cups escarole or spinach, torn in bite-size pieces (1/2 head)
3 hard-cooked eggs, cut in quarters

Antipasto Dressing:
1 (6-oz.) jar marinated artichoke hearts, undrained
1/4 cup red wine vinegar
2 garlic cloves, pressed or minced
2 tablespoons chopped parsley
1/2 teaspoon dried oregano
1/4 teaspoon pepper
3 flat anchovy fillets, rinsed, drained, chopped

Prepare Antipasto Dressing; cover and let stand for 2 hours for flavors to blend. In a large salad bowl, layer tuna, broccoli, cherry tomatoes, radishes, olives, bell pepper, onion, romaine and escarole. If assembled ahead, cover and refrigerate for up to 2 hours. Pour dressing over salad; toss gently to mix. Garnish with egg quarters. Makes 6 main-dish salads.

Antipasto Dressing:
In a small bowl, combine artichoke hearts and their liquid, wine vinegar, garlic, parsley, oregano, pepper and anchovies; stir gently to combine.

PER SERVING: 1/6 of total recipe				
CALORIES	CARBOHYDRATES	PROTEIN	FAT	CHOLESTEROL
172	10 gm	15 gm	8 gm	139 mg

Taco Salad

For an easy dinner that is short on fat and long on flavor, you can't beat this high protein salad. Make the baked tortilla bowls a day ahead, if you like, and store airtight in a large plastic bag. Start the meal with refreshing Blender Gazpacho, page 69, and offer Fruit & Berry Gratin, page 175, as a sweet conclusion.

4 (8-inch) whole wheat *or* regular flour tortillas
2/3 lb. lean ground chuck
1 small onion, chopped (3 oz.)
1 garlic clove, pressed *or* minced
1 (15-oz.) can kidney beans, drained, rinsed
1-1/2 teaspoons chili powder
1/4 teaspoon ground cumin
1 (8-oz.) can tomato sauce
4 cups finely sliced iceberg *or*
    leaf lettuce (1 small head)
1/2 cup shredded Cheddar cheese (2 oz.)
2 tablespoons sliced pitted ripe olives
1/4 cup low-fat sour cream
2 green onions, thinly sliced, including tops
1 medium-size tomato, cut into 8 wedges (5 oz.)
4 green pepperoncini

Preheat oven to 350F (175C). Cut 8 (9-inch) circles of heavy duty foil. Place 4 circles on work surface; top each with another foil circle. Heat a large skillet over medium heat. One at a time, warm tortillas in skillet 30 seconds on each side or until soft and pliable. Place each warm tortilla on a set of foil circles. Bring edges of foil up so tortillas become bowl-shaped approximately 5 inches across the bottom and with flaring sides. Place tortilla bowls, in their foil molds, on 2 ungreased baking sheets. Bake 1 sheet in preheated oven for 12 minutes or until tortillas are crisp and lightly browned. Remove from oven. Repeat with remaining sheet. Let cool completely before lifting tortilla bowls from foil molds. Heat a large skillet over medium-high heat. Crumble in meat; cook until browned. Add onion and garlic; reduce heat to medium. Cook until onion is soft but not browned; drain and discard drippings. Add beans, chili powder, cumin and tomato sauce. Simmer, uncovered, for 10 minutes or until mixture thickens slightly. To assemble salads, place tortilla bowls on 4 individual plates. Fill each bowl with 1 cup of lettuce. Top each with an equal amount of hot meat mixture, cheese, and olives. Place 1 tablespoon sour cream atop each salad; sprinkle with green onions. Garnish each salad with 2 tomato wedges and 1 pepperoncini. Makes 4 main-dish salads.

PER SERVING: 1/4 of total recipe				
CALORIES	**CARBOHYDRATES**	**PROTEIN**	**FAT**	**CHOLESTEROL**
445	48 gm	30 gm	15 gm	67 mg

Chinese Chicken Salad

This dinner-size Oriental chicken salad is higher in protein and lower in fat than most versions. An added advantage: Instead of deep-frying bean threads for the traditional garnish, you soften soup noodles in the sweet-spicy dressing. Look for Chinese plum sauce packed in bottles or cans in the Oriental section of your market.

Plum Sauce Dressing (recipe below)
1 (3-oz.) package Oriental noodle soup mix
3 tablespoons slivered almonds
2 tablespoons sesame seeds
2-1/2 cups shredded cooked chicken breast
4 green onions, thinly sliced, including tops
4 cups finely sliced iceberg lettuce (1 small head)
1/2 cup cilantro leaves, coarsely chopped

Plum Sauce Dressing:
1/4 cup Chinese plum sauce
1-1/2 tablespoons sugar
1-1/2 tablespoons white wine vinegar
1 teaspoon lemon juice
1 tablespoon pineapple juice *or* orange juice
1 tablespoon vegetable oil
2 teaspoons sesame oil
1 teaspoon dry mustard
Salt to taste

Prepare Plum Sauce Dressing; set aside. Open package of noodle soup mix; discard seasoning packet. Crumble noodles into a small bowl. Add half of dressing; mix well. Let stand, covered, at room temperature for 45 minutes or until noodles soften slightly. Place almonds in a small dry skillet over medium heat. Toast, stirring often, for 3 minutes or until golden. Place almonds in a large salad bowl. Place sesame seeds in dry skillet. Toast, over low heat, shaking skillet frequently, for 2 minutes or until seeds turn golden and begin to pop. Add to almonds, along with chicken, green onions, lettuce, cilantro and softened noodles and their dressing. Pour remaining dressing over salad. Toss to coat evenly. Makes 4 main-dish salads.

Plum Sauce Dressing:
In a medium-size bowl, combine plum sauce, sugar, wine vinegar, lemon juice, pineapple juice, vegetable oil, sesame oil, dry mustard and salt to taste; whisk to blend evenly. If made ahead, cover and refrigerate up to 3 days. Makes about 1/2 cup.

PER SERVING: 1/4 of total recipe

CALORIES	CARBOHYDRATES	PROTEIN	FAT	CHOLESTEROL
355	23 gm	31 gm	16 gm	71 mg

Low-Cal Herb Dressing

This all-purpose dressing shines when it dresses a salad accented with fruit. Try it with raw spinach tossed with thinly sliced apple or Mandarin oranges; sliced oranges, sliced red onion, jicama, and slivers of avocado; or mixed greens tumbled with cubes of fresh pear and seedless grapes. Compared to commercially prepared Italian Salad Dressing, this low-calorie dressing has 64 fewer calories and 6 grams less of fat.

1/4 cup olive oil
2 tablespoons white wine vinegar
2 tablespoons lemon juice
1 (6-oz.) can vegetable juice cocktail
1 tablespoon Dijon-style mustard
1 tablespoon chopped parsley
1 tablespoon chopped chives
1/2 teaspoon dried basil
Dash red (cayenne) pepper
1 garlic clove, pressed *or* minced

In a pint jar, with a lid, combine oil, wine vinegar, lemon juice, vegetable juice cocktail, mustard, parsley, chives, basil, red pepper and garlic. Cover jar; shake until dressing is blended. Use at once or refrigerate for up to 1 week. Bring to room temperature and shake again before adding to a salad. Makes 1-1/3 cups.

PER SERVING: 1 tablespoon				
CALORIES	CARBOHYDRATES	PROTEIN	FAT	CHOLESTEROL
25	1 gm	0 gm	3 gm	0 mg

Creamy Yogurt Dressing

Spoonful for spoonful, this easily-made dressing has half the amount of fat of blue cheese or ranch dressing. It's the perfect way to showcase summer's produce: juicy tomatoes, crisp cucumber slices, thinly sliced raw mushrooms or crisp-cooked green beans.

1/4 cup olive oil
1/4 cup cider vinegar
1-1/2 teaspoons Dijon-style mustard
1-1/2 teaspoons lemon juice
1 small garlic clove, cut in half
1/4 teaspoon dried dill
1/4 cup plain low-fat yogurt
1/2 teaspoon sugar
Salt and pepper to taste

In a blender, combine oil, vinegar, mustard, lemon juice, garlic, dill, yogurt and sugar. Process until smooth and creamy. Add salt and pepper to taste. Pour into a jar with a lid. Cover; refrigerate for up to 4 days. Makes about 1 cup.

PER SERVING: 1 tablespoon				
CALORIES	CARBOHYDRATES	PROTEIN	FAT	CHOLESTEROL
38	1 gm	0 gm	4 gm	0 mg

Thousand Island Dressing

You'd swear this was rich with mayonnaise, but it's not. Use it for your favorite crab or shrimp Louie, a whole meal tuna or chicken salad or as a creamy topping for crisp hearts of lettuce.

1/2 cup low-fat sour cream
1/4 cup ketchup
1 teaspoon Dijon-style mustard
1/2 teaspoon prepared horseradish
1 large green onion, finely minced, white part only
3 tablespoons finely chopped dill pickle
1 hard-cooked egg, finely chopped
White pepper to taste

In a small bowl, combine sour cream, ketchup, mustard and horseradish; whisk until smooth. Stir in green onion, dill pickle, chopped egg and pepper to taste. Cover and refrigerate for up to 3 days. Makes 1 cup.

PER SERVING: 1 tablespoon

CALORIES	CARBOHYDRATES	PROTEIN	FAT	CHOLESTEROL
14	2 gm	1 gm	1 gm	18 mg

Storing Salad Greens:
If you have washed salad greens on hand, you are more likely to make a salad when time is short. Wash greens as soon as you get home from the market. Spin them dry in a salad spinner or pat them dry with paper towels. Put in a large plastic bag and store in the crisper of your refrigerator. These will keep, if well dried, for 3 or 4 days.

BREADS

Bread is a nutritious part of a balanced diet, and it is especially important for the active person. It supplies energy for muscles and many of the B vitamins which are very important for energy conversion. Historically, bread in many cuisines has supplied a majority of the daily calories, however, today we have often neglected this nutrient-rich food in our diets. For optimum health chose a selection of fiber-rich whole-grain breads.

In this chapter, you'll find breads with a variety of flavors and fanciful shapes. Some of the recipes in this chapter use the food processor for a speedy mix of ingredients, but you'll also find make-by-hand instruction if a food processor is not available.

You can prepare any of the muffin recipes, cool completely then wrap in foil and freeze. When time is short on a week-day morning, remove a muffin from foil, then just pop one of these little gems in the microwave, placed on a paper towel, on High for 15 seconds for a quick meal on the run.

No-Knead Dilly Bread, opposite, bakes in a loaf pan so you can slice it for sandwiches. Puffy Broiler Bread, page 167, is a round that puffs up to make a pocket. Banana Bran Muffins, page 170, taste like cupcakes. Unlike most muffins which taste best hot, these little breads are good cold—a great pick-me-up with mid-morning coffee. Cranberry Orange Bread, page 172, is sweet enough to stand in for dessert, and would be a nice accompaniment to a chicken or turkey salad. Pancakes, another form of "bread," are covered in the Breakfast & Brunch chapter.

No one bread is perfect, nor is any one bread bad when eaten occasionally. It's just that some choices are wiser than others in terms of fat content and calories.

	FAT (gm)	CALORIES
1 bagel	1	163
1 Danish, plain	9	161
1 English muffin	1	135
1 doughnut, yeast-raised	8	124
1 croissant	6	109
1 slice French bread	1	70
1 slice whole-wheat bread	1	61
2 graham crackers, 2-inch squares	1.5	60
2 rye crackers, triple crackers	0	50
1 rice cake	0	30

No-Knead Dilly Bread

This moist, flavorful bread is especially high in thiamin. Made with quick-rising yeast, this loaf calls for a different mixing technique than the one used with conventional yeast. Use a thermometer to determine the temperature of the liquid mixture so yeast will react. If you use an egg directly from the refrigerator, place it in a small bowl and cover with warm tap water for 5 minutes to bring to room temperature.

3 tablespoons instant minced onion
1-1/2 cups whole-wheat flour
1-1/4 cups all-purpose flour
1 (1/4-oz.) pkg. quick-rising yeast (*about* 1 tablespoon)
2 tablespoons sugar
2 teaspoons dried dill
1 teaspoon salt
2 tablespoons margarine
1/2 cup water
1 cup plain low-fat yogurt
1 egg, room temperature

Grease a 9″ x 5″ loaf pan with vegetable nonstick cooking spray. Sprinkle 1 tablespoon of the onion evenly over bottom of pan; set aside. In a large bowl, combine remaining 2 tablespoons onion, whole-wheat flour, 1/2 cup of the all-purpose flour, yeast, sugar, dill and salt; stir until evenly mixed. In a saucepan, heat margarine over medium heat until melted. Add water and yogurt; whisk until smooth. Heat mixture to 125F (50C), or until hot to the touch. Stir into flour mixture. Stir in egg, then remaining 3/4 cup all-purpose flour to make a stiff batter. Spoon into prepared pan; spread in an even layer. Place pan in a 13″ x 9″ pan half filled with hottest tap water. Cover both pans with a dry cloth towel. Let rise in a draft-free place for 30 minutes or until almost doubled in bulk. Preheat oven to 375F (190C). Remove loaf pan from water bath. Bake in preheated oven 30 minutes or until loaf is nicely browned and sounds hollow when tapped. Cool on a wire rack 10 minutes; turn bread out onto rack to cool completely. Makes 16 (1/2-inch) slices.

PER SERVING: 1/2-inch slice

CALORIES	CARBOHYDRATES	PROTEIN	FAT	CHOLESTEROL
109	19 gm	4 gm	2 gm	17 mg

Wheaty Peanut Butter Buns

Add a little protein to your diet with these surprise filled rolls. They make a hearty accompaniment to soups or salads, and are quick to make in the food processor. To intensify the natural sweetness of the peanut butter filling, serve these buns warm or reheated.

1/4 cup warm water (110F/45C)
1 (1/4-oz.) pkg. active dry yeast (*about* 1 tablespoon)
1-1/4 cups all-purpose flour
1-1/4 cups whole-wheat flour
1/2 teaspoon salt
1 tablespoon sugar
1/4 cup water
1/2 cup skim milk
2 tablespoons plus 1 teaspoon vegetable oil
1/4 cup chunky peanut butter

Pour warm water into a small bowl; sprinkle yeast over water and stir until dissolved. Let stand 10 minutes or until small bubbles form. In a food processor, combine all-purpose flour, whole-wheat flour, salt and sugar; process 10 seconds. In a 1-cup glass measure, combine water, milk and 2 tablespoons of the oil. With food processor running, pour milk mixture down the feed tube, then pour dissolved yeast down the feed tube. Process just until mixture forms a ball. On a lightly floured surface, knead dough 5 minutes or until smooth and elastic. Grease a large bowl with the remaining 1 teaspoon oil. Place dough in bowl; turn to coat. Cover bowl with a dry cloth towel; let rise in a warm, draft-free place for 1-1/4 hours or until doubled in bulk. Punch dough down; knead 1 minute. Divide dough into 12 equal-size pieces. Shape each piece into a flat circle about 4 inches in diameter; press outer edge of circle to make it slightly thinner than the center. Place 1 teaspoon peanut butter in center of each round. Draw edges of dough up and around filling; twist to seal. Grease a large shallow baking pan with vegetable nonstick cooking spray. Place buns, sealed-side-down, 2 inches apart, in pan. Cover and let rise in a warm place 45 minutes or until puffy and light. Preheat oven to 350F (175C). Bake in preheated oven 15 minutes or until tops are golden brown. Serve warm or cool on a wire rack. To reheat, place on a pan in 350F oven for about 10 minutes or until warm to the touch. Makes 12 buns.

To make dough by hand:
Combine dry ingredients in a large bowl. Make a well in the center; add milk mixture and dissolved yeast. Stir with a heavy wooden spoon until dough forms a ball. On a lightly floured surface, knead dough 10 minutes or until smooth and elastic. Proceed with instructions above for rising, shaping and baking.

PER SERVING: 1 bun

CALORIES	CARBOHYDRATES	PROTEIN	FAT	CHOLESTEROL
142	21 gm	5 gm	5 gm	0 mg

Puffy Broiler Bread

Made with ease and speed, this chewy bread is high in B vitamins. These bread rounds are delicious served with soup or fruit salad. Or, you can also cut each round in half to hold a sandwich filling. Watch the bread closely as it broils; once it puffs and begins to brown, it cooks very quickly.

> 2 cups all-purpose flour
> 1-1/2 teaspoons baking powder
> 1 teaspoon sugar
> 1/2 teaspoon salt
> 1/8 teaspoon baking soda
> 1 egg
> 1/2 cup skim milk
> 3 tablespoons plain low-fat yogurt
> 1 tablespoon margarine, melted
> 1 teaspoon poppy seeds

In a food processor, combine flour, baking powder, sugar, salt and baking soda; process for 30 seconds. In a small bowl, whisk egg lightly. Add milk and yogurt; whisk until evenly blended. With processor running, pour egg mixture down the feed tube. Continue to process until mixture forms a ball. Remove dough and knead 1 minute or until smooth and elastic. Grease a bowl with 1 teaspoon of the margarine. Place dough in bowl; turn to coat. Cover bowl with a dry cloth towel; let rest for 45 to 60 minutes (dough will not rise.) Divide dough into 8 equal-size pieces. Roll each piece into a ball. With fingertips, press each ball into a circle about 4 inches in diameter, 1/8-inch thick in the center, and no more than 1/4-inch thick on the edges. Rub 1/4 teaspoon margarine over top of each dough circle; sprinkle lightly with poppy seeds. Preheat broiler. Place 2 or 3 pieces of bread, poppy-seed-side-up, on an ungreased baking sheet. Broil 6 inches from heat, 2 minutes or until bread puffs and turns golden. Turn over and continue to broil 1 to 2 more minutes or until golden. Remove bread puffs to a wire rack; cool 5 minutes before serving. Repeat with remaining bread puffs. Makes 8 servings.

To make dough by hand:
Combine dry ingredients in a medium-size bowl. Make a well in the center; pour in egg-milk mixture. Stir until well blended. Turn dough onto a smooth surface; knead 10 minutes or until smooth and elastic. Proceed with instructions above for resting, shaping and broiling.

PER SERVING: 1 bread puff

CALORIES	CARBOHYDRATES	PROTEIN	FAT	CHOLESTEROL
150	26 gm	5 gm	2 gm	35 mg

Grilled Garlic Bread

A tasty, garlicky toast technique adopted from Italy, this garlic bread can also be toasted under the broiler. Here is a good reason to splurge on extra-virgin olive oil. Made from the first pressing of high-quality ripe olives, extra-virgin olive oil has an intense fruity flavor and marries well with garlic.

> **1/2 long loaf sweet *or* sourdough French *or***
> **Italian bread (half 1-lb. loaf) *or* 1 baguette (8 oz.)**
> **2 garlic cloves, cut in half**
> **3 tablespoons extra-virgin olive oil**
> **Salt to taste (optional)**

Cut bread in half lengthwise; cut each half crosswise into 4 pieces. Rub cut side of bread with cut side of garlic. Place bread, cut-side-down on a grill 4 to 6 inches above a solid bed of low-glowing coals. Lightly toast until bread begins to turn golden with insides of bread somewhat soft. Or, toast bread under a preheated broiler. Immediately brush bread with olive oil. Sprinkle with salt, if desired. Serve warm. Makes 8 servings.

PER SERVING: 1/8 of total recipe				
CALORIES	**CARBOHYDRATES**	**PROTEIN**	**FAT**	**CHOLESTEROL**
124	16 gm	3 gm	5 gm	0 mg

Savory Popovers

Served piping hot from the oven, these flavorful shells make any soup or salad seem special. If you choose ham as the flavor enhancer, be sure to trim off any visible fat before using.

> **1 tablespoon yellow cornmeal**
> **1 cup all-purpose flour**
> **1/4 teaspoon salt**
> **2 eggs**
> **1 cup skim milk**
> **1 tablespoon margarine, melted, cooled**
> **1 (4-oz.) can diced green chiles *or* 1/2 cup**
> **minced cooked lean ham**

Preheat oven to 400F (205C). Grease a muffin pan with 2-1/2-inch diameter cups with vegetable nonstick cooking spray. Dust each cup with about 1/4 teaspoon of cornmeal; set aside. In a medium-size bowl, combine flour and salt; stir until evenly mixed. In a separate bowl, beat eggs; stir in milk and margarine. Add egg mixture to dry ingredients. With an electric mixer or rotary beater, beat until very smooth. Pour 1 tablespoon batter into each prepared muffin cup. Place 2 teaspoons chiles on top of batter in each cup. Fill cups 2/3 full with remaining batter. Bake in preheated oven 35 minutes or until well browned and firm to the touch. Remove from pan; serve hot. Makes 12 popovers.

PER SERVING: 1 popover				
CALORIES	**CARBOHYDRATES**	**PROTEIN**	**FAT**	**CHOLESTEROL**
90	11 gm	5 gm	3 gm	49 mg

Whole-Wheat Millet Muffins

Millet gives these muffins an intriguingly crunchy texture as well as generous amounts of essential amino acids, B vitamins, phosphorous and iron. Mildly sweet, they can substitute nicely for bread at dinner. Look for millet in health-food stores.

1 cup all-purpose flour
3/4 cup whole-wheat flour
1/4 cup whole millet
3 tablespoons sugar
1/2 teaspoon salt
1 tablespoon baking powder
1 egg, lightly beaten
1 cup skim milk
1/4 cup margarine, melted, cooled

Preheat oven to 400F (205C). Grease a muffin pan with 2-1/2-inch diameter cups with vegetable nonstick cooking spray; set aside. In a medium-size bowl, combine all-purpose flour, whole-wheat flour, millet, sugar, salt and baking powder; stir until evenly mixed. Make a well in center of dry ingredients. In a separate bowl, combine egg, milk and margarine; whisk to evenly blend. Pour into dry ingredients; stir just until dry ingredients are moistened (do not beat). Fill each prepared muffin cup 2/3 full with batter. Bake in preheated oven 15 to 20 minutes or until tops are lightly browned. Remove muffins from pan to a wire rack; cool 5 minutes. Serve warm. Makes 12 muffins.

PER SERVING: 1 muffin

CALORIES	CARBOHYDRATES	PROTEIN	FAT	CHOLESTEROL
136	20 gm	4 gm	5 gm	20 mg

Saving Time With Muffins:
Muffins and quick breads take only minutes to whip up, but you may want to get a head start the night before. Prepare pan. Measure dry ingredients into a mixing bowl, cover, and keep on the kitchen counter. In the morning, measure liquid ingredients, combine the two and pop your breads into the oven.

Apple-Oatmeal Muffins

Lightly spiced with cinnamon and chunky apple bits, these muffins are a wholesome addition to any breakfast. This recipe makes plenty for another meal; freeze the cooled extra muffins in foil. Another day when time is short, pull one of these high-fiber muffins from the freezer, place on a paper towel and warm it in the microwave on High for 15 seconds.

> 1-1/2 cups quick-cooking oatmeal
> 1 cup all-purpose flour
> 1/4 cup sugar
> 3/4 teaspoon salt
> 2-1/2 teaspoons baking powder
> 1/2 teaspoon baking soda
> 1/2 teaspoon ground cinnamon
> 1 egg, lightly beaten
> 1 cup skim milk
> 2 tablespoons vegetable oil
> 1 1/2 cup finely chopped, cored, peeled apple (8 oz.)

Preheat oven to 400F (205C). Grease a muffin pan with 2-1/2-inch diameter cups with vegetable nonstick cooking spray; set aside. Place oatmeal in a blender; process 2 minutes or until oats resemble coarse flour. In a medium-size bowl, combine processed oatmeal, flour, sugar, salt, baking powder, baking soda and cinnamon; stir until evenly mixed. Make a well in center of dry ingredients. In a separate bowl, combine egg, milk and oil; whisk to evenly blend. Pour into dry ingredients; stir just until dry ingredients are moistened (*do not beat*). Stir in apple until evenly distributed. Fill each prepared muffin cup 2/3 full with batter. Bake in preheated oven 15 to 20 minutes or until a wooden pick inserted in center comes out clean. Remove muffins from pan to a wire rack; cool 5 minutes. Serve warm or cool completely. Any extra muffins can be wrapped in foil and frozen. Makes 16 muffins.

PER SERVING: 1 muffin				
CALORIES	CARBOHYDRATES	PROTEIN	FAT	CHOLESTEROL
110	19 gm	3 gm	3 gm	15 mg

Banana Bran Muffins

Here's a way to add fiber to your breakfast. Enjoy this nutrient-dense bread with a glass of grapefruit or orange juice for a quick breakfast on the run.

> 1/2 cup skim milk
> 2/3 cup whole-bran cereal
> 1/4 cup sugar
> 2 tablespoons vegetable oil
> 1 egg, lightly beaten
> 1 cup all-purpose flour
> 1 teaspoon baking powder
> 1/2 teaspoon baking soda
> 1/2 teaspoon salt
> 2 bananas, peeled, thinly sliced (2 cups)

Preheat oven to 375F (190C). Grease a muffin pan with 2-1/2-inch diameter cups with vegetable nonstick cooking spray; set aside. In a small pan, heat milk to scalding; remove pan from heat. Add cereal; stir to moisten. When cool, add sugar, oil and egg; mix well. Into a medium-size bowl, sift flour, baking powder, baking soda and salt. Make a well in center; add cereal mixture. Stir just until ingredients are blended (batter will be rather stiff). Add bananas; stir until fruit is evenly distributed. Fill each prepared muffin cup 2/3 full with batter. Bake in preheated oven 25 minutes or until tops are lightly browned. Remove muffins from pan to a wire rack; cool 5 minutes. Serve warm or cool completely. Makes 12 muffins.

PER SERVING: 1 muffin

CALORIES	CARBOHYDRATES	PROTEIN	FAT	CHOLESTEROL
108	19 gm	2 gm	3 gm	20 mg

Baked Brown Bread

This iron-rich bread, paired with baked beans, tastes wonderful on a cold day. Serve it plain or lavish it with spicy apple butter.

1/2 cup all-purpose flour
1/2 cup whole-wheat flour
1/2 cup yellow cornmeal
1 teaspoon baking soda
1/2 teaspoon salt
1/2 cup raisins
1 cup buttermilk *or* sour milk, *or* 3/4 cup plus 2 tablespoons
   skim milk combined with 2 tablespoons cider vinegar
1/3 cup molasses
1 tablespoon margarine, melted, cooled

Preheat oven to 350F (175C). Grease an 8-1/2" x 4-1/2" loaf pan with vegetable nonstick cooking spray; set aside. In a medium-size bowl, combine all-purpose flour, whole-wheat flour, cornmeal, baking soda and salt; stir until evenly mixed. Add raisins; stir to coat. In a separate bowl, combine buttermilk, molasses and margarine; whisk to evenly blend. Pour into dry ingredients; stir until dry ingredients are moistened. Pour batter into prepared pan. Bake in preheated oven 35 minutes or until a wooden pick inserted in center comes out clean. Cool in pan on a wire rack for 10 minutes. Turn loaf out onto rack. Cut warm bread with serrated knife. Makes 16 (1/2-inch) slices.

Variation: To make Boston-Style Steamed Brown Bread, grease a 1-pound coffee can with vegetable nonstick cooking spray. Pour in batter. Cover top of can with a double layer of foil; shape foil to fit can top snugly. Place can in a deep kettle with a lid; add boiling water to kettle until it comes halfway up the can side. Cover kettle; steam for 1-1/2 hours or until a wooden pick inserted in center comes out clean. Remove from kettle. Cool on wire rack 10 minutes. Serve warm. Makes 16 (1/2-inch) slices.

PER SERVING: 1/2-inch slice

CALORIES	CARBOHYDRATES	PROTEIN	FAT	CHOLESTEROL
85	18 gm	2 gm	1 gm	0 mg

Cranberry Orange Bread

Here's a great way to include complex carbohydrates for a snack, or as an accompaniment to a fruit salad or a turkey dinner. If you use frozen cranberries, rinse them in a colander, then chop in a food processor while still frozen.

    2 cups whole-wheat flour
    1/4 cup non-fat dry milk powder
    1 teaspoon baking powder
    1 teaspoon baking soda
    1/2 teaspoon salt
    1/4 cup margarine, room temperature
    2/3 cup honey
    2 eggs
    1 cup orange juice
    1/2 cup chopped walnuts
    2 cups whole cranberries, fresh *or* frozen, coarsely chopped

Preheat oven to 350F (175C). Grease a 9" x 5" loaf pan with vegetable nonstick cooking spray; set aside. In a large bowl, combine flour, dry milk powder, baking powder, baking soda and salt; stir until evenly mixed. In a medium-size bowl, stir margarine and honey together until creamy; add eggs, one at a time, stirring well after each addition. Stir in orange juice. Pour into dry ingredients; stir until dry ingredients are moistened. Stir in walnuts and cranberries. Spoon batter into prepared pan. Bake in preheated oven 1 hour or until a wooden pick inserted in center comes out clean. Cool, in pan, on wire rack 10 minutes. Turn loaf out onto rack; cool completely. Store leftover bread in a plastic bag at room temperature for 2 days or freeze for later use. Makes 16 (1/2-inch) slices.

PER SERVING: 1/2-inch slice

CALORIES	CARBOHYDRATES	PROTEIN	FAT	CHOLESTEROL
169	27 gm	4 gm	6 gm	35 mg

Banana Apricot Bread

Tuck this energy booster into your pack to take on a long bike ride or day hike. It's delicious plain or sandwiched with ricotta cheese.

    1/2 cup dried apricots
    1 cup all-purpose flour
    1 cup whole-wheat flour
    1 teaspoon baking powder
    1 teaspoon baking soda
    1/4 teaspoon salt
    1/4 cup margarine, softened
    2/3 cup packed brown sugar
    1 egg
    1 teaspoon grated orange peel
    1/4 cup orange juice
    2 medium-size bananas, pureed (1 cup)

Preheat oven to 350F (175C). Grease a 9'' x 5'' loaf pan with vegetable nonstick cooking spray; set aside. In a small bowl, cover apricots with hot water; let stand 10 minutes. Drain apricots; finely chop. In a large bowl, combine all-purpose flour, whole-wheat flour, baking powder, baking soda and salt; stir until evenly mixed. In a medium-size bowl, cream margarine and brown sugar; beat in egg. Stir in orange peel, orange juice and bananas. Pour into dry ingredients; stir until dry ingredients are moistened. Stir in apricots. Spoon batter into prepared pan. Bake in preheated oven 1 hour or until a wooden pick inserted in center comes out clean. Cool, in pan, on wire rack 10 minutes. Turn loaf out onto rack; cool completely. Store leftover bread in a plastic bag at room temperature for up to 2 days or freeze for later use. Makes 16 (1/2-inch) slices.

PER SERVING: 1/2-inch slice

CALORIES	CARBOHYDRATES	PROTEIN	FAT	CHOLESTEROL
139	26 gm	3 gm	4 gm	17 mg

Date Bran Bread

This bread is nutrient-dense for all nutrients except vitamin C. Pair it with a sunshine fruit—an orange or grapefruit—for a quick breakfast, or enjoy it as an after-dinner sweet.

3/4 cup plus 2 tablespoons whole-wheat flour
1 cup all-purpose flour
1/4 cup wheat germ
1/3 cup packed brown sugar
1 tablespoon baking powder
1 teaspoon ground cinnamon
2/3 cup chopped, pitted dates
2 eggs
1-1/3 cups skim milk
2 tablespoons molasses
2 tablespoons margarine, melted, cooled
1-1/4 cups whole-bran cereal

Preheat oven to 350F (175C). Grease a 9'' x 5'' loaf pan with vegetable nonstick cooking spray; set aside. In a large bowl, combine whole-wheat flour, all-purpose flour, wheat germ, brown sugar, baking powder and cinnamon; stir until evenly mixed. Add dates; mix with your hands until date pieces are separated and coated with flour. In a medium-size bowl, whisk eggs slightly. Add milk, molasses and margarine; whisk until well blended. Stir in whole bran cereal. Pour into dry ingredients; stir until dry ingredients are moistened. Spoon batter into prepared pan. Bake in preheated oven 1 hour or until a wooden pick inserted in center comes out clean. Cool, in pan, on wire rack 10 minutes. Turn loaf out onto rack; cool completely. Store leftover bread in a plastic bag at room temperature for up to 2 days or freeze for later use. Makes 16 1/2-inch slices.

PER SERVING: 1/2-inch slice

CALORIES	CARBOHYDRATES	PROTEIN	FAT	CHOLESTEROL
139	27 gm	4 gm	3 gm	35 mg

DESSERTS

You can have your cake and good health too, if you eat cake only occasionally, then choose one, which is low in fat and calories. Keeping fit does not mean denying your sweet tooth, but it does call for making the right choices.

For day-to-day sweets, nothing can compete with fruit. Fruits are nutrient bargains. They supply large amounts of vitamins, minerals and fiber with small numbers of calories. Today, you don't even have to shop a specialty market to find an array of fresh fruit year round.

What happens when you tire of eating fresh fruit out of hand? In this chapter you'll find light, easy fruit recipes such as Fruit & Berry Gratin, opposite, or Creamy Berry Ice, page 178, for a change of pace. Strawberry Cheesecake Crepes, page 181, and Apple Strudel, page 183, are perfect for those times when you want a show-stopper dessert.

Is dessert, for you, a final act to *every* meal? If so, try a slice of angel food cake or sponge cake topped with fresh fruit or canned fruit packed in its own juice. Or try walking instead. Walking boosts energy, relieves tension and gives your brain a chance to "register" that you are full. It takes about 20 minutes for the satisfied feeling signal to reach your brain. When there is a time lapse between dinner and dessert, you will be a little less hungry and a piece of fresh fruit will be as fulfilling as the thought of a piece of double chocolate layer cake.

Fruit & Berry Gratin

Fifteen minutes is all you need to whip up this brown-sugar crusted gratin. Broil it just before serving dinner; it's best served slightly warm.

        1-1/2 cups raspberries *or* blueberries
        1/2 cup low-fat sour cream
        1-1/2 cups peeled, sliced peaches, nectarines *or*
            fresh figs, cut in half
        1 tablespoon Cointreau *or* other orange flavored liqueur
            (optional)
        1/3 cup packed brown sugar

Evenly place berries in a 1-quart souffle dish or other ovenproof dish that measures 6 to 7 inches in diameter. Spread sour cream over berries. Arrange peaches in an even layer over sour cream. Sprinkle with liqueur. Sprinkle brown sugar in an even layer over fruit. Preheat broiler. Broil 3 to 4 inches from heat for 2 minutes or until sugar melts evenly but does not burn. Remove to a wire rack. Let cool 15 minutes before serving. Makes 6 servings.

PER SERVING: 1/6 of total recipe

CALORIES	CARBOHYDRATES	PROTEIN	FAT	CHOLESTEROL
96	21 gm	1 gm	1 gm	2 mg

Strawberries & Peaches in Wine

Here is a great way to toast a win. Serve this dessert-beverage combination in large wine glasses, then sip the wine after spooning out the fruit.

        2 cups strawberries, hulled
        2 cups sliced, peeled, fresh *or* unsweetened frozen peaches
        1/2 cup sugar
        1/2 cup orange juice
        1 teaspoon grated orange peel
        1 tablespoon lemon juice
        1/4 cup Port wine *or* sweet vermouth
        1/2 cup dry white wine

In a large bowl, place strawberries, peaches, sugar, orange juice, orange peel and lemon juice. (If using frozen peaches, let mixture stand at room temperature until peaches thaw.) Stir gently to mix. Pour Port and white wine over fruit. Cover and refrigerate for up to 1 hour or for as long as 4 hours. With a slotted spoon evenly divide fruit into 6 large wine glasses. Add fruit-liquid to each glass. Makes 6 servings.

PER SERVING: 1/6 of total recipe

CALORIES	CARBOHYDRATES	PROTEIN	FAT	CHOLESTEROL
217	46 gm	1 gm	0 gm	0 mg

Fruit Compote with Raspberry Sauce

Do you think of fiber as a breakfast filler-upper? One serving of this baked compote has as much fiber as 2-2/3 cups of bran flake cereal. It's a fine way to end a wintry meal for two.

1 large banana, peeled, cut in half lengthwise then
   crosswise (8 oz.)
1 large pear, quartered, cored, peeled (8 oz.)
8 pitted prunes
1/2 cup dry red wine
1/2 cup fresh *or* frozen unsweetened raspberries, thawed
1/2 cup orange juice
2 tablespoons honey
1/2 teaspoon grated lime peel

Place banana, pear, prunes, and wine in a plastic bag; seal bag. Refrigerate for 8 hours. Pour off wine; if desired, save for other uses. Place fruit in a quiche dish or 1-quart casserole. In a food processor or blender, combine raspberries, orange juice and honey. Process until pureed. Pour over fruit. Bake, uncovered, in a 350F (175C) oven for 20 minutes. Remove from oven to a wire rack; let stand until cool. Just before serving, sprinkle with lime peel. Makes 2 servings.

PER SERVING: 1/2 of total recipe				
CALORIES	CARBOHYDRATES	PROTEIN	FAT	CHOLESTEROL
257	60 gm	2 gm	1 gm	0 mg

Poached Plums with Apple Snow

Prepare this refreshing fruity dessert on the weekend for a delicious mid-week treat.

1 lb. plums, pitted, cut in quarters
3 tablespoons sugar
2 tablespoons water
1 cinnamon stick (3 inches)
2 whole cloves

Apple Snow:
1-1/2 teaspoons unflavored gelatin
2/3 cup cold water
1/3 cup frozen apple juice concentrate

Place plums in a medium-size saucepan. Add sugar, water, cinnamon stick and cloves. Stirring, bring to a boil over high heat. Reduce heat; cover and simmer 6 to 8 minutes or until plums are fork-tender when pierced. Remove from heat; let cool. Pour into a container with a tight fitting lid; cover. Refrigerate for up to 3 days. Prepare Apple Snow. To serve, spoon Apple Snow into 4 serving bowls. Place plums beside snow. Discard cinnamon and cloves. Dividing juices evenly, pour over plums and snow. Makes 4 servings.

Apple Snow:
In a small sauce pan, stir gelatin into water; let stand 3 minutes to soften. Stir over low heat just until gelatin dissolves. Remove from heat; stir in apple juice concentrate. Pour into a medium-size bowl. Place bowl in a larger bowl of ice water; stir occasionally until mixture mounds slightly when dropped from a spoon, about 15 minutes. With electric mixer, beat snow until frothy. Cover and refrigerate until firm, for up to 2 hours or for as long as 3 days.

PER SERVING: 1/4 of total recipe				
CALORIES	CARBOHYDRATES	PROTEIN	FAT	CHOLESTEROL
130	32 gm	2 gm	0 gm	0 mg

Grapefruit Meringue Shells

Whoever would have guessed that a breakfast staple could look so glamorous? This supplies your day's requirement for vitamin C.

2 large pink *or* white grapefruit (12 oz. *each*)
2 egg whites, room temperature (1/4 cup)
1/4 cup sugar
2 tablespoons sweetened flaked coconut

Preheat oven to 300F (150C). Cut grapefruit in half crosswise. Place a sieve over a bowl and set aside. With a serrated grapefruit spoon or knife, remove sections of fruit between membranes. Drop into sieve; discard seeds. When all fruit is removed, gently squeeze shells over sieve so juice drains through sieve. Let fruit drain. With the spoon, scrape out all pulp from shells so only white part remains. In a small bowl of an electric mixer, beat egg whites until frothy. Add sugar, 1 tablespoon at a time, beating well after each addition. Continue beating until meringue holds glossy, stiff peaks. With a rubber spatula, fold well drained grapefruit segments into meringue. Spoon meringue into grapefruit shells. Sprinkle coconut evenly over top of shells. Place shells in a shallow baking pan. Bake in preheated oven for 20 minutes or until meringue is lightly browned. Remove shells to a wire rack and let cool for at least 15 minutes, but no longer than 1 hour because meringue will begin to weep. Makes 4 servings.

PER SERVING: 1/2 grapefruit				
CALORIES	CARBOHYDRATES	PROTEIN	FAT	CHOLESTEROL
146	33 gm	3 gm	1 gm	0 mg

Spicy Poached Pears

Year-round enjoyment is yours with this luscious low-fat dessert. You can make it with either summer Bartlett pears or one of the winter varieties, such as Bosc, Comice or d'Anjou.

2 large pears, halved, cored, peeled (8 oz. *each*)
1 cup apple cider
1 teaspoon lemon juice
1 cinnamon stick (3 inches)
5 whole cloves
6 dates, pitted, thinly sliced
2 tablespoons low-fat sour cream
1/8 teaspoon ground nutmeg

Place pears in a medium-size saucepan. Add cider, lemon juice, cinnamon stick and cloves. Bring to a boil over medium heat; reduce heat. Cover; simmer 8 to 10 minutes or until pears are tender when pierced. With a slotted spoon remove pear halves to 4 dessert bowls; cored side up. Add dates to pan juices. Bring to a boil over medium heat. Boil, uncovered, 5 minutes or until juices thicken slightly; discard cinnamon stick and cloves. Dividing sour cream equally, spoon into pear core cavities. Spoon date sauce over each pear. Sprinkle each with nutmeg. Serve warm or chilled. Makes 4 servings.

PER SERVING: 1/4 of total recipe				
CALORIES	**CARBOHYDRATES**	**PROTEIN**	**FAT**	**CHOLESTEROL**
143	36 gm	1 gm	1 gm	1 mg

Creamy Berry Ice

This tangy refreshing ice is very simple to make and it is as luscious as it is light and cool. You can make it with frozen berries if you want to bring the taste of summer to a mid-winter meal.

2/3 cup water
1/2 cup sugar
2 cups unsweetened raspberries, blackberries *or*
    boysenberries, thawed if frozen
1 tablespoon lemon juice
2 tablespoons Creme de Cassis, blackberry liqueur *or*
    thawed orange juice concentrate
2 egg whites, room temperature

In a small saucepan, heat water and sugar until sugar dissolves; let cool. In a large bowl, crush berries with a potato masher or process in a food processor until pureed. Place a sieve over a medium-size bowl. Pour crushed berries through sieve. Smash with the back of a spoon to release as much juice as possible; discard seeds. Stir cooled sugar syrup, lemon juice, and liqueur into juice. In a small bowl, beat egg whites until they hold stiff peaks; fold into berry mixture. Pour into a 9-inch square pan. Freeze for 2 hours or until firm. With a fork, break mixture into small pieces; transfer to a food processor fitted with a metal blade or the large bowl of an electric mixer. Beat until smooth and slushy. Spoon into a 1-quart container with a lid. Cover and freeze until firm, about 3 hours, or for up to 2 weeks. Let stand at room temperature 5 minutes before serving. Makes 6 (1/2-cup) servings.

PER SERVING: 1/2 cup				
CALORIES	CARBOHYDRATES	PROTEIN	FAT	CHOLESTEROL
104	25 gm	1 gm	0 gm	0 mg

Strawberry Sorbet

Keep this cooling, slightly tart ice on hand in your freezer for a pause that refreshes after a long hard workout. Serve it in a cone or be elegant and serve it in a pretty glass bowl. Because of the alcohol in the Cointreau, this sorbet freezes but won't become crystalized.

> 4 cups strawberries, hulled
> 1 cup orange juice
> 1/4 cup lemon juice
> 1-1/4 cups sugar
> 1/4 cup Cointreau *or* other orange-flavored liqueur (optional)
> 2 egg whites, room temperature

In a food processor or blender, combine strawberries, orange juice and lemon juice; process until pureed. Pour into a large bowl. Add 1 cup of the sugar and liqueur. Let stand 30 minutes, stirring occasionally, until sugar dissolves. After sugar dissolves, in a medium-size bowl, beat egg whites until frothy. Add the remaining 1/4 cup sugar, 1 tablespoon at a time, beating well after each addition. Continue beating until meringue holds glossy, stiff peaks. With a wire whisk, fold meringue into strawberry mixture. Pour into a 13″ x 9″ pan. Freeze for 2 or 3 hours or until firm. With a fork, break mixture into small pieces; transfer a portion at a time to a food processor fitted with a metal blade or the large bowl of an electric mixer. Beat until smooth and slushy. Spoon into a 2-quart container with a lid. Cover and freeze until firm, about 3 hours, or for up to 2 weeks. Let stand at room temperature 5 minutes before serving. Makes 14 (1/2 cup) servings.

PER SERVING: 1/2 cup				
CALORIES	CARBOHYDRATES	PROTEIN	FAT	CHOLESTEROL
102	24 gm	1 gm	1 gm	0 mg

Pineapple-Lime Sherbet

Icy cold and tart-sweet, this refreshing sherbet gains its creamy quality from low-fat buttermilk. If you don't use buttermilk as a beverage, look for the pint-size carton of buttermilk in the dairy section of your market.

1 (6-oz.) can frozen pineapple juice concentrate, thawed
1/3 cup sugar
1/2 cup lime juice
1 teaspoon grated lime peel
2 cups buttermilk

In a medium-size saucepan, combine pineapple juice and sugar. Heat over medium heat until sugar dissolves. Remove from heat; let cool. Add lime juice, lime peel and buttermilk; mix well. Pour into 2 divided ice cube trays; freeze for 1-1/2 to 2 hours or until almost firm. Transfer cubes to a food processor fitted with a metal blade or the large bowl of an electric mixer. Beat until smooth and slushy. Spoon into a 1-quart container with a lid. Cover and freeze until firm, about 3 hours, or for up to 2 weeks. Let stand at room temperature 5 minutes before serving. Makes 8 (1/2-cup) servings.

PER SERVING: 1/2 cup

CALORIES	CARBOHYDRATES	PROTEIN	FAT	CHOLESTEROL
93	21 gm	2 gm	1 gm	2 mg

Cheesecake Mousse

This dessert is light and luscious. At 140 calories per serving, you can have your cake and eat it too.

1 (1/4-oz.) envelope unflavored gelatin (about 1 tablespoon)
1/2 cup cold skim milk
1 egg, separated
1-1/2 cups low-fat cottage cheese
1/4 cup thawed, frozen unsweetened orange juice concentrate
4 tablespoons sugar
1 teaspoon grated lemon peel
2 tablespoons lemon juice
5 fresh mint sprigs *or* 5 small strawberries

In a small pan, stir gelatin into cold milk; let stand 3 minutes to soften. Stir over low heat just until gelatin dissolves. Remove from heat and let cool until warm to the touch. In a blender, combine egg yolk, cottage cheese, orange juice concentrate, 2 tablespoons of the sugar, lemon peel and lemon juice. Add gelatin mixture. Process 2 minutes or until very smooth. Pour into a medium-size bowl. Place bowl in a larger bowl of ice water; stir occasionally until mixture mounds slightly when dropped from a spoon, about 15 minutes. Remove bowl from ice water. In a small bowl, quickly beat egg white until frothy. Beat in remaining 2 tablespoons sugar, 1 tablespoon at a time, beating well after each addition. Continue beating until meringue holds glossy, stiff peaks. Fold meringue into cheese mixture. Dividing mousse equally, spoon into 5 dessert dishes. Refrigerate until firm, for up to 3 hours or for as long as 24 hours. To serve, garnish each serving with a mint sprig or strawberry. Makes 5 servings.

PER SERVING: 1/5 of total recipe				
CALORIES	CARBOHYDRATES	PROTEIN	FAT	CHOLESTEROL
140	18 gm	12 gm	2 gm	60 mg

Strawberry Cheesecake Crepes

You don't need to tell your family or friends they are getting their day's requirement of vitamin C with this luscious dessert. Just serve these strawberry-topped crepes and let them feel properly pampered.

> 2/3 cup part-skim ricotta cheese
> 1/3 cup Neufchâtel cheese, softened
> 2 tablespoons thawed, frozen orange juice concentrate
> 1 teaspoon grated lemon peel
> 8 Crepes (page 187)
> 3 cups strawberries, hulled, sliced
> 1 tablespoon sugar
> 1 teaspoon lemon juice

In a food processor, combine ricotta cheese, Neufchâtel cheese, orange juice concentrate and lemon peel; process until creamy. Grease a 13" x 9" baking pan with vegetable nonstick cooking spray; set aside. To fill crepes: place one crepe, brown-side down, on work surface. Place 2 tablespoons of cheese filling across lower 1/3; roll to enclose. Place filled crepe, seam-side-down, in prepared pan. Repeat with remaining crepes and filling. If assembled ahead, cover and refrigerate up to 24 hours. One hour before serving, combine strawberries, sugar, and lemon juice in a bowl. Let stand at room temperature for 1 hour or until berries are juicy. Preheat oven to 350F (175C). Bake crepes, uncovered, for 15 minutes or until filling is warm and edges of crepes are golden brown (20 minutes if refrigerated). To serve, place 2 crepes on each of 4 plates. Spoon strawberries over each serving. Makes 4 servings.

PER SERVING: 2 crepes				
CALORIES	CARBOHYDRATES	PROTEIN	FAT	CHOLESTEROL
173	19 gm	8 gm	8 gm	26 mg

Spicy Apple Cake

Here is comfort food with homemade goodness. Each serving has less fat than a teaspoon of margarine. After the cake cools, if you wish, cut it in serving-size portions, pack in plastic sandwich bags and freeze for quick lunch treats.

> 1/4 cup vegetable oil
> 3/4 cup sugar
> 1 egg
> 1 teaspoon vanilla extract
> 1 cup all-purpose flour
> 1 teaspoon baking soda
> 1/4 teaspoon salt
> 1 teaspoon ground cinnamon
> 1/4 teaspoon ground nutmeg
> 1/8 teaspoon ground ginger
> 1/8 teaspoon ground allspice
> 2 cups chopped, peeled, cored, apples, Golden Delicious *or*
>   Newtown Pippin (1 lb.)
> 1/2 cup raisins

Preheat oven to 350F (175C). Grease an 8-inch square baking pan with vegetable nonstick cooking spray; set aside. In a large bowl, combine oil and sugar; add egg and mix well. Stir in vanilla. Sift flour, baking soda, salt, cinnamon, nutmeg, ginger and allspice into sugar mixture. Stir until well blended (batter will be stiff). Add apples and raisins. Stir just until fruit is evenly distributed. Spoon batter into prepared pan; spread with rubber spatula to make an even layer. Bake in preheated oven 30 minutes or until a wooden pick inserted in center comes out clean. Remove pan from oven; place on a wire rack. Cool 30 minutes before cutting. Makes 16 (2-inch) servings.

PER SERVING: 1 (2-inch) square

CALORIES	CARBOHYDRATES	PROTEIN	FAT	CHOLESTEROL
128	23 gm	2 gm	4 gm	16 mg

Apple Strudel

Instead of serving apples in a pie, try them in this plump juicy strudel. You trim both fat and calories when you use a filo wrapper in place of a pastry crust. Filo comes in 1-pound packages in the refrigerator or freezer section of your grocery store. If filo is frozen, let unopened package thaw in the refrigerator. For this recipe remove the 3 sheets filo just before assembling strudel. Keep covered with a dry dish towel to prevent from drying out. Return the unused portion to a plastic bag; close tightly and store in the refrigerator for up to 3 weeks or in the freezer for up to 6 months.

5 cups thinly sliced apples, Golden Delicious *or* Newtown
    Pippin (3 medium-size apples)
1/2 cup granulated sugar
1/4 cup finely chopped walnuts
1 teaspoon lemon juice
1/2 teaspoon ground cinnamon
1/8 teaspoon ground ginger
1/8 teaspoon ground nutmeg
3 sheets filo
3 tablespoons margarine, melted
1/3 cup unseasoned dry bread crumbs
1 tablespoon powdered sugar

Preheat oven to 375F (190C). Line a 15″ x 10″ jelly-roll pan with foil; set aside. In a large bowl, combine apples, granulated sugar, walnuts, lemon juice, cinnamon, ginger and nutmeg; stir gently. Place 1 sheet of filo on a clean tea towel. Brush in streaks with 1/4 of the margarine. Sprinkle with half of the bread crumbs. Repeat, using 1 more sheet of filo, 1/4 of the margarine and the remaining bread crumbs. Top with a third sheet of filo. Streak with half of the remaining margarine. Spoon apple filling and any juices along one long side, 2 inches from filo edge. Fold long edge up part way over filling. Using the towel to help you lift, roll up loosely jelly-roll fashion. Using towel, lift strudel to pan; gently slide into pan, seam-side-down. Ends of filo will remain open. Prick top of filo with a fork in 3 or 4 places. Brush remaining margarine over sides and top of strudel. Bake in preheated oven for 35 minutes or until golden brown. Let cool until slightly warm; cut in 6 portions. Dust each serving lightly with powdered sugar. Strudel tastes best if served within 3 hours after cooling otherwise it becomes too soggy. Makes 6 servings.

PER SERVING: 1/6 of total recipe				
CALORIES	CARBOHYDRATES	PROTEIN	FAT	CHOLESTEROL
228	36 gm	3 gm	8 gm	0 mg

Using Filo:
If filo is frozen, let the unopened package thaw overnight in the refrigerator. For easiest handling, let fresh or thawed, frozen filo stand at room temperuature, unopened for two hours before using.

Almond Cookie Shells

Almonds are high in fat, but a few of them go a long way to give sweetness and crunchiness to this crisp-edged cookie shell. A scoop of sherbet, sorbet or an ice makes a delicious filling. Or you may prefer to fill the shells with seasonal fruit, such as a mixture of raspberries, blueberries and sliced peaches. Then dust lightly with powdered sugar. Do not use a blender to grind almonds because it blends them into too fine a powder.

      3 tablespoons blanched almonds (1 oz.)
      2 tablespoons all-purpose flour
      2 tablespoons sugar
      1/4 cup egg whites, room temperature (2 egg whites)

Preheat oven to 350F (175C). Grease a baking sheet with vegetable nonstick cooking spray; set aside. Place almonds in a pie pan. Bake in preheated oven for 8 to 10 minutes or until lightly toasted; let cool. Very finely chop almonds in a food processor or grate with a rotary grater. In a small bowl, combine almonds, flour and sugar. In a medium-size bowl, whisk egg whites until frothy. Stir in almond mixture. Bake 2 cookies at a time. For each cookie, place 1-1/2 tablespoons of batter, about 6 inches apart, on prepared baking sheet. With a spatula, spread batter to make a 5-inch circle. Bake in preheated oven 10 to 12 minutes or until a 1 inch band around edge of cookies is golden brown and centers are light brown. Immediately loosen cookies from sheet with a spatula; drape each cookie over a glass that measures about 2 inches across the bottom. Protecting your hands with pot holders, gently press cookies around 2 glasses to form flat-bottomed cups with flaring sides. As soon as cookies hold their shape, about 1 minute, transfer to a wire rack and cool completely. Repeat, using the remainder of the batter. Use shells at once, or store airtight, at room temperature, for up to 2 days. Fill with suggested fillings above. Makes 4 cookie shells.

PER SERVING: 1 cookie shell				
CALORIES	CARBOHYDRATES	PROTEIN	FAT	CHOLESTEROL
86	11 gm	3 gm	4 gm	0 mg

Chocolate Kisses

You can savor this chocolate treat and be free of calories, fat and guilt. Two cookies contain fewer calories than one 4-inch graham cracker.

      1/4 cup powdered sugar
      1-1/2 tablespoons unsweetened cocoa powder
      2 egg whites, room temperature (1/4 cup)
      1/3 cup granulated sugar
      1/4 teaspoon vanilla extract
      2 cups four-grain cereal flakes

Preheat oven to 300F (150C). Grease a baking sheet with vegetable nonstick cooking spray; set aside. Into a medium-size bowl, sift powdered sugar and cocoa. In a large bowl of an electric mixer, beat egg whites until frothy. Add granulated sugar, 1 tablespoon at a time, beating well after each addition. Continue beating until meringue holds glossy, stiff peaks. Beat in vanilla. Sprinkle powdered sugar-cocoa mixture over meringue. With a rubber spatula, fold the two mixtures just until evenly blended. Add cereal flakes; fold gently until flakes are coated with meringue. Drop meringue mixture, 2 teaspoons for each cookie, 1 inch apart, onto prepared baking sheet. Bake in preheated oven for 20 minutes or until outside of each cookie is dry and set. Let cool on baking sheet 5 minutes; transfer to racks to cool completely. Store in an airtight container. Makes 28 cookies.

PER SERVING: 1 cookie

CALORIES	CARBOHYDRATES	PROTEIN	FAT	CHOLESTEROL
22	20 gm	2 gm	0 gm	0 mg

Oatmeal-Raisin Bars

It's nice to know that a cookie can taste good and be good for you as well. This quickly-made bar is low in fat and provides generous amounts of vitamin A, thiamin and iron.

> 1-1/2 cups quick-cooking rolled oats
> 1/4 cup non-fat dry milk powder
> 1 cup all-purpose flour
> 1/2 teaspoon baking powder
> 1/2 teaspoon baking soda
> 1/2 teaspoon ground cinnamon
> 1/2 teaspoon salt
> 1 cup raisins
> 1/4 cup water
> 1/3 cup vegetable oil
> 1/3 cup molasses *or* honey
> 1 cup sliced carrot (1 medium-size)
> 1/2 cup firmly packed brown sugar
> 1 egg

Preheat oven to 350F (175C). Grease a 13" x 9" baking pan with vegetable nonstick cooking spray; set aside. In a large bowl, combine oats, milk powder, flour, baking powder, baking soda, cinnamon, salt and raisins; stir until evenly mixed. Make a well in the center. In a blender, combine water, oil, molasses and carrot; process until carrot is very finely chopped. Add brown sugar and egg; process 30 seconds. Pour into dry ingredients. Stir until dry ingredients are well moistened. Pour batter into prepared pan; spread with rubber spatula to make an even layer. Bake in preheated oven 30 minutes or until a wooden pick inserted in center comes out clean. Remove pan from oven; place on a wire rack. Cool in pan 30 minutes. Cut into bars. Makes 24 (2"x 1-1/2") bars.

PER SERVING: 1 (2" x 1-1/2") bar

CALORIES	CARBOHYDRATES	PROTEIN	FAT	CHOLESTEROL
117	20 gm	2 gm	3 gm	10mg

BREAKFAST & BRUNCH

It's not nutritionally smart to save calories by skipping breakfast. Blood sugar is low after an all-night fast, and the body needs refueling so it can work at peak performance. Ironically, breakfast skippers usually make up for the "saved" calories later in the day—typically before bed.

Whatever the morning brings, don't fall into the too-late-for breakfast trap. Ideally, breakfast should include fruit or juice that contains vitamin C; one-third of the day's protein which can come from low-fat yogurt or milk, cottage cheese or an occasional egg; and a complex carbohydrate such as whole-grain bread or cereal. For starters, try Quick Banana Milkshake, page 197, or Creamy Tofu Cooler, page 197, made in seconds with the whirl of a blender. Corn Griddle Cakes, page 191, or Cinnamon-Apple Pancakes, page 190, are so tempting you may want to get up early to try them. For more ideas on complex carbohydrates, turn to the chapter on Breads.

On weekends, when there is time for a leisurely breakfast or brunch, relax and enjoy Portuguese Breakfast Eggs, page 193, or Crab-Filled Crepes, page 188. Egg dishes are high in cholesterol and it's best to limit your egg intake to three or four a week. Don't forget to count the eggs contained in baked products.

Because of their high saturated fat content, breakfast meats do not make a championship breakfast. If you want to keep your muscle and lose fat, eat these meats no more than one to two times a week. A diet rich in saturated fat and cholesterol is identified as a major risk factor for coronary heart disease. Stick with the low-fat meats, such as Canadian bacon or turkey sausage, and serve them in 2-ounce portions. Most breakfast meats have a salty, intense flavor so a little goes a long way. Look for low-sodium products if you are on a sodium-reduced diet.

Crepes

These tender pancakes make a thin wrapper for either a sweet or savory filling. Swirl the batter as soon as it is placed in the hot pan: don't worry if there are one or two tiny holes where the batter did not completely cover the pan surface. They will never be noticed once the crepe is rolled up. Turning the crepes over is easiest when you use a pan with a nonstick finish.

> 2 eggs
> 1-1/2 cups skim milk
> 1 cup all-purpose flour
> 1 tablespoon vegetable oil
> 4-1/2 teaspoons margarine

In a blender or food processor, combine eggs, milk, flour and oil. Process until smooth. Pour batter into a small bowl. Let rest at room temperature 1 hour or cover and refrigerate overnight. Place a 6- or 7-inch crepe pan or other flat-bottom nonstick frying pan over medium-high heat. When hot, add 1/4 teaspoon of the margarine; swirl to coat surface. Stir batter; pour 2 tablespoons batter into center of pan. Quickly tilt pan in all directions so batter flows over entire flat surface. Cook until surface is dry and edge is lightly browned. Turn crepe over; cook 10 seconds. Turn crepe out of pan onto a paper towel. Repeat procedure with remaining batter, using 1/4 teaspoon of margarine to grease pan before making each crepe. When cool, stack crepes and use within a few hours. To keep longer, place waxed paper between each crepe, seal in an airtight package and refrigerate up to 3 days or freeze for longer storage. Allow crepes to come to room temperature before separating; they will tear if they are still cold. Makes 18 (6-inch) crepes.

Variation Dessert Crepe: If you plan to fill crepes with a sweet filling, add 1 teaspoon vanilla to crepe batter.

PER SERVING: 1 crepe

CALORIES	CARBOHYDRATES	PROTEIN	FAT	CHOLESTEROL
58	6 gm	2 gm	3 gm	31 mg

Crab-Filled Crepes

Here's proof that healthy food can be festive. Serve this make-ahead entree for brunch, lunch or dinner accompanied with steamed asparagus and fresh fruit salad.

1-1/2 tablespoons margarine
1 tablespoon minced onion
1-1/2 tablespoons all-purpose flour
1 cup low-fat milk
1 tablespoon grated Parmesan cheese
1/2 teaspoon dried dill
1/2 lb. crabmeat *or* surimi-style (imitation) crabmeat, flaked
10 Crepes (page 187)
5 tablespoons Butterless Hollandaise Sauce (page 194)

In a small skillet melt margarine over medium heat. Add onion; cook until onion is soft but not browned. Stir in flour; cook 1 minute or until bubbly. Remove pan from heat. Gradually stir in milk. Return pan to heat. Stirring constantly, cook until sauce is smooth and thickened. Stir in Parmesan cheese. Remove skillet from heat. Add dill and crabmeat; stir gently. Grease a 13" x 9" baking pan with vegetable nonstick cooking spray; set aside. To fill crepes, place crepes, browned-side-down, on work surface. Place 2 tablespoons of crab mixture across lower 1/3 of each crepe; roll to enclose. Place filled crepes, seam-side-down, in prepared pan. If assembled ahead, cover and refrigerate up to 24 hours. Preheat oven to 350F (175C). Bake crepes, uncovered, 15 minutes (20 minutes if refrigerated) or until filling is hot and edges of crepes are golden brown. Warm hollandaise sauce as directed in recipe on page 195. To serve, place 2 crepes on each plate. Spoon 1 tablespoon hollandaise sauce over each serving. Makes 5 servings.

PER SERVING: 2 crepes				
CALORIES	CARBOHYDRATES	PROTEIN	FAT	CHOLESTEROL
245	17 gm	15 gm	13 gm	145 mg

Bircher Muesli

About the same time that Dr. John Harvey Kellogg devised Corn Flakes to improve the health of his sanitarium patients in Battlecreek, Michigan, Dr. R. Bircher-Benner was looking for ways to improve the diets of his patients in his clinic in Zurich. The result was Bircher Museli. The Swiss accepted this dish of uncooked oatmeal, milk and fruits with such gusto that today it is known as a national dish in Switzerland. It is nutritionally balanced and a tasty way to start the day.

> 1/3 cup quick-cooking oatmeal
> 1 tablespoon raisins
> 1/3 cup low-fat milk
> 1 medium-size apple, peeled, cored (5 oz.)
> 1 tablespoon lemon juice
> 1 tablespoon honey
> 1 tablespoon chopped almonds *or* walnuts

Place oatmeal and raisins in a large cereal bowl; pour in milk. Let stand 20 minutes or cover and refrigerate overnight. To serve, grate apple over cereal. Add lemon juice, honey and nuts. Makes 1 serving.

PER SERVING: 1 bowl

CALORIES	CARBOHYDRATES	PROTEIN	FAT	CHOLESTEROL
345	67 gm	8 gm	8 gm	5 mg

Ricotta Cheese Pancakes
with Strawberries

This easy breakfast for two is loaded with vitamin C and protein.

> 1-1/2 cups strawberries, hulled, sliced
> 1 tablespoon sugar
> 1/2 teaspoon lemon juice
> 1/2 cup part-skim ricotta cheese (4 oz.)
> 1 egg
> 1/3 cup skim milk
> 1/4 cup all-purpose flour
> 1/2 teaspoon baking powder
> Salt to taste

In a medium-size bowl, combine strawberries, sugar and lemon juice; stir until well mixed. Set aside. In a food processor or blender combine ricotta cheese and egg; process 1 minute. Add milk, flour, baking powder and salt; process until smooth. Preheat a griddle or large skillet over medium heat; grease with vegetable nonstick cooking spray. Spoon 2 tablespoons batter onto griddle for each pancake; spread out to 3-inch circles. Cook until edges appear dry; turn and cook other side until golden brown. Remove from griddle and keep warm. Cook remaining pancakes. Spoon strawberries mixture over pancakes. Makes 8 pancakes.

PER SERVING: 4 pancakes with strawberries

CALORIES	CARBOHYDRATES	PROTEIN	FAT	CHOLESTEROL
262	33 gm	14 gm	9 gm	159 mg

Cinnamon-Apple Pancakes

Whether your goal is to load up on carbohydrates or just get a good start for the day, here is a way to do it with fiber and flavor. Top these cinnamon pancakes with warm apple butter and turn them into a truly nutritious breakfast.

    1/3 cup all-purpose flour
    2/3 cup whole-wheat flour
    1 teaspoon baking powder
    1/4 teaspoon baking soda
    2 teaspoons sugar
    1/2 teaspoon salt
    1/4 teaspoon ground cinnamon
    1/8 teaspoon ground nutmeg
    1/4 cup wheat germ
    1 whole egg plus 1 egg white
    1 cup buttermilk *or* 2 tablespoons distilled white vinegar
      mixed with 3/4 cup plus 2 tablespoons skim milk
    1 Granny Smith *or* Golden Delicious apple, peeled, shredded
      (1 cup)

In a sifter over a medium-size bowl, combine all-purpose flour, whole-wheat flour, baking powder, baking soda, sugar, salt, cinnamon and nutmeg; sift. Stir in wheat germ and make a well in the center. In a separate bowl, whisk together the whole egg and the egg white. Add buttermilk; whisk until blended. Pour liquid into well; stir just until dry ingredients are moistened. Stir in apple. Preheat a griddle or large skillet over medium heat; grease with vegetable nonstick cooking spray. Spoon about 1/4 cup batter onto griddle for each pancake; spread batter out to make 4-inch circles. Cook until tops of pancakes are bubbly and appear dry; turn and cook other side until browned. Makes 15 pancakes.

PER SERVING: 3 pancakes				
CALORIES	CARBOHYDRATES	PROTEIN	FAT	CHOLESTEROL
187	34 gm	8 gm	3 gm	54 mg

Oven-Baked Pancake with Glazed Fruit

You don't want a late-arriving guest when you serve this showy brunch dish. Straight from the oven, the pancake is puffed and billowy; but after 5 minutes it begins to collapse. Serve it with glasses of chilled pineapple juice.

    3 eggs
    3/4 cup skim milk
    3/4 cup all-purpose flour
    1/8 teaspoon salt
    3 tablespoons margarine
    1 cup seedless grapes
    2 medium-size oranges, peeled, cut in bite-size pieces
    1 tablespoon sugar
    1/4 teaspoon ground cinnamon

Preheat oven to 425F (220C). In a food processor or blender, combine eggs and milk; process until well mixed. Add flour and salt; process until smooth. Place 2 tablespoons of the margarine in a 1-1/2-quart ovenproof casserole. Place casserole in preheated oven 4 minutes or until margarine melts and bubbles. Remove casserole from oven; pour batter into melted margarine. Return casserole to oven; bake 20 minutes or until pancake is puffy and edges are golden brown. Just before pancake is done, in a medium-size skillet melt remaining 1 tablespoon margarine over medium heat. Add grapes and oranges; cook 2 minutes. Add sugar and cinnamon; cook 1 minute or until fruit is glazed. As soon as pancake is removed from the oven, cut into 4 wedges and spoon glazed fruit over each serving. Makes 4 servings.

PER SERVING: 1/4 of total recipe

CALORIES	CARBOHYDRATES	PROTEIN	FAT	CHOLESTEROL
307	39 gm	9 gm	13 gm	184 mg

Corn Griddle Cakes

Start your day with a taste of the South: sliced peaches, corn-filled griddle cakes splashed with warm maple syrup and a slice of Canadian bacon. It adds up to a breakfast that is high in B vitamins and fiber.

1/2 cup all-purpose flour
1/2 cup yellow cornmeal
2 teaspoons baking powder
1 tablespoon sugar
1/2 teaspoon salt
1 egg
1 cup skim milk
2 tablespoons vegetable oil
1 cup cooked corn or 1 (8-oz.) can whole kernel corn,
    drained well

In a medium-size bowl, combine flour, cornmeal, baking powder, sugar and salt; stir until well mixed. In a separate bowl, whisk egg slightly. Add milk and oil; whisk until blended. Pour liquid into dry ingredients; stir just until flour and cornmeal are moistened. Stir in corn. Preheat a griddle or large skillet over medium heat; grease with vegetable nonstick cooking spray. Scooping batter from bottom of bowl, spoon 3 tablespoons batter onto griddle for each pancake. Spread batter out to make 4-inch circles. Cook until tops of pancakes are bubbly and appear dry; turn and cook other sides until browned. Makes 16 pancakes.

PER SERVING: 4 pancakes

CALORIES	CARBOHYDRATES	PROTEIN	FAT	CHOLESTEROL
259	38 gm	8 gm	9 gm	62 mg

Mushroom Potato Pie

As an alternative to quiche, try this easy, crustless vegetable pie that can be prepared well in advance and then baked when you are ready. For a summer brunch, serve it with papaya halves filled with fresh raspberries and blueberries.

4 medium-size thin-skinned boiling potatoes (1 lb. *total*)
1 teaspoon margarine
1/4 lb. mushrooms, sliced
2 tablespoons regular-strength chicken broth
1/2 teaspoon salt
1/4 teaspoon pepper
1/2 teaspoon caraway seeds
3 eggs
1 cup low-fat cottage cheese (8 oz.)
2 tablespoons lemon juice
4 drops hot pepper sauce
1/4 teaspoon paprika

In a medium-sized saucepan, cook unpeeled potatoes in 2 inches boiling water 25 minutes or until fork-tender; drain. Set potatoes aside until cool enough to handle. Peel cooked potatoes; cut in 1/4-inch-thick slices. In a large skillet melt margarine over medium heat. Add mushrooms and chicken broth. Increase heat to high. Cook 5 minutes or until all liquid evaporates and mushrooms just begin to turn golden. Preheat oven to 350F (175C). Grease a 9-inch pie pan with vegetable nonstick cooking spray. Place half the potatoes in bottom of pie pan; cover with half the mushrooms. Sprinkle with half the salt, pepper and caraway seeds. Repeat, making another layer. In a blender, combine eggs, cottage cheese, lemon juice and hot pepper sauce. Process until very smooth. If making the night before, cover and refrigerate egg mixture and vegetable mixture separately. Pour mixture evenly over vegetable layers. Sprinkle paprika over top. Bake in preheated oven 30 minutes or until pie is puffed and golden brown and a knife inserted in center comes out clean. Cool in pan on a wire rack for 5 minutes before cutting. Makes 6 servings.

PER SERVING: 1/6 of total recipe

CALORIES	CARBOHYDRATES	PROTEIN	FAT	CHOLESTEROL
136	16 gm	9 gm	4 gm	125 mg

Portuguese Breakfast Eggs

After running the par-course, pat yourself on the back and enjoy a lazy Sunday breakfast. Squeeze a wedge of lime over honeydew melon for starters. Savory Popovers, page 168, would taste good with these eggs. If you wish to double the recipe, use a 12-inch skillet.

2 tablespoons olive oil
1 medium-size onion, chopped (5 oz.)
1 garlic clove, pressed *or* minced
1 lb. zucchini, diced
1 small green bell pepper, seeded, cored, chopped (4 oz.)
1 tablespoon chopped parsley
1 tablespoon chopped celery leaves
1/2 cup tomato sauce
1/2 teaspoon dried basil
1/2 teaspoon dried oregano
3 eggs
1/4 cup skim milk
1/4 teaspoon salt
1/8 teaspoon pepper
1/4 cup shredded Longhorn *or* mild Cheddar cheese (1 oz.)

In a 10-inch skillet heat oil over medium-high heat. Add onion, garlic, zucchini, bell pepper, parsley and celery leaves. Cook, stirring occasionally, for 5 minutes. Reduce heat to medium-low; cover skillet. Continue to cook 5 more minutes or until zucchini is crisp-tender. Add tomato sauce, basil and oregano. Simmer, uncovered, 5 minutes or until sauce thickens slightly. In a small bowl, combine eggs, milk, salt and pepper; whisk until evenly blended. Pour over zucchini mixture. Cover skillet; cook 5 minutes or until eggs are set but still moist on the top. Sprinkle cheese evenly over eggs. Preheat broiler. Place skillet 6 inches under broiler; broil 1 minute or until cheese melts. Cut in 4 wedges and serve from the skillet. Makes 4 servings.

PER SERVING: 1/4 of total recipe

CALORIES	CARBOHYDRATES	PROTEIN	FAT	CHOLESTEROL
204	14 gm	9 gm	13 gm	192 mg

Nash's Chili Egg Puff

Quick, easy and delicious, this chile-laced casserole is good for breakfast, lunch or dinner. Serve it with fresh fruit, a green salad or sauteed mixed vegetables and crusty French bread. It is a good source of calcium, riboflavin and vitamin C.

> 1/4 cup all-purpose flour
> 1/2 teaspoon baking powder
> 1/4 teaspoon salt
> 5 eggs
> 1 cup low-fat cottage cheese
> 1 cup shredded farmer *or* Cheddar cheese (4 oz.)
> 1 (4-oz.) can diced green chilies
> 1 tablespoon margarine

Preheat oven to 350F (175C). In a small bowl, combine flour, baking powder and salt; stir to blend. In a large bowl, beat eggs until frothy. Stir in cottage cheese, farmer cheese and green chilies; stir until well mixed. Place margarine in an 8-inch-square baking pan. Place pan in preheated oven 4 minutes or until margarine melts and bubbles. Remove pan from oven and pour batter into melted margarine. Return pan to oven and bake 35 minutes or until a knife inserted in center comes out clean. Let stand on a wire rack 5 minutes before cutting in squares. Makes 6 servings.

PER SERVING: 2 tablespoons				
CALORIES	CARBOHYDRATES	PROTEIN	FAT	CHOLESTEROL
34	5 gm	3 gm	0 gm	1 mg

Butterless Hollandaise Sauce

It's no wonder classic hollandaise is not an everyday sauce. The egg-butter blend is too rich to be eaten with any frequency. This low-fat version of hollandaise is a smashing choice to accent eggs, salmon, asparagus or artichokes. The more vigorously you whip the sauce during cooking, the greater the volume.

> 3 eggs, room temperature
> 3 tablespoons lemon juice
> 3 tablespoons regular-strength chicken broth
> 1 teaspoon Dijon-style mustard
> 1/4 teaspoon salt
> Red (cayenne) pepper to taste

Using a wire whisk, combine eggs, lemon juice and chicken broth in the top of a double boiler. Pour hot water into bottom of double boiler, making sure water won't touch bottom of top pan. Bring water to a boil over high heat; reduce heat to keep water at a simmer. Set top pan in place over bottom of double broiler. Whisk mixture vigorously and constantly for 4 minutes or until sauce is thick and fluffy. As soon as sauce thickens, remove top pan. Whisk in mustard, salt and red pepper to taste. Serve immediately. Or, if made ahead, pour into a jar. When cool, cover and refrigerate up to 3 days. To reheat, place jar in a pan of water that is hot to the touch; stir until sauce is warm but not hot. Makes 1-1/3 cups.

PER SERVING: 1 tablespoon

CALORIES	CARBOHYDRATES	PROTEIN	FAT	CHOLESTEROL
11	0 gm	1 gm	1 gm	35 mg

Eggs Benedict

Splurge and enjoy it. But don't do it frequently and do cut back on your cholesterol intake for the rest of the day. For the average person, the daily recommendation is 300 mg of cholesterol. It is not heart-healthy to overstep this limit on a regular basis. Accompany with tall glasses of orange juice and melon wedges.

> **1/3 lb. Canadian bacon, sliced 1/8 to 1/4 inch thick**
> **3 English muffins, halved**
> **Butterless Hollandaise Sauce (opposite)**
> **1 tablespoon distilled white vinegar *or* cider vinegar**
> **6 eggs**

In a wide skillet, cook bacon over medium heat until lightly browned and heated through; keep warm. Toast muffin halves. Reheat hollandaise sauce as directed above. Pour water into a wide skillet to a depth of 1-1/2 inches; add vinegar. Heat just until small bubbles form on bottom of pan. Break each egg into the water, keeping each one separate. With water barely simmering, cook eggs until done to your liking: For soft yolks and firm whites, allow 3 to 5 minutes. Remove eggs with a slotted spoon and place on paper towels to drain. To serve, place 1 muffin half on each plate. Cover each with a bacon slice. Place 1 egg on each bacon-topped muffin half; spoon 1 tablespoon hollandaise sauce over each egg. Makes 6 servings.

PER SERVING: 1/6 of total recipe

CALORIES	CARBOHYDRATES	PROTEIN	FAT	CHOLESTEROL
215	14 gm	15 gm	11 gm	302 mg

Huevos Rancheros

Here's another classic breakfast dish which is best eaten on days when your remaining meals will be low in cholesterol. You can cook the Mexican-style eggs two ways: Poach them in salsa and serve them right from the skillet, or bake them with salsa in ramekins for individual servings. Serve with refried beans, warm tortillas and skewered fresh fruit for a winning, hearty brunch.

2 teaspoons vegetable oil
1 small onion, chopped (3 oz.)
1 large garlic clove, pressed *or* minced
1 (16-oz.) can whole peeled tomatoes
1/4 cup canned diced green chiles
1/4 teaspoon ground cumin
1/4 teaspoon dried oregano
Salt to taste
6 eggs
6 tablespoons shredded Cheddar cheese (1-1/2 oz.)
6 cilantro sprigs

In a large skillet heat oil over medium heat. Add onion and garlic; cook until onion is soft but not browned. Pour tomatoes with their liquid into skillet; coarsely cut up tomatoes. Add green chilies, cumin and oregano. Simmer, uncovered, 10 minutes or until salsa is slightly thickened. Add salt to taste. If poaching the eggs, make 6 wells in salsa with the back of a spoon. Break an egg into each well. Sprinkle 1 tablespoon cheese over each egg. Cover skillet; cook 5 minutes or until eggs are set to your liking. Serve from the skillet; garnish each serving with a sprig of cilantro. If baking the eggs, preheat oven to 350F (175C). Divide salsa evenly among 6 (10-ounce) ramekins or custard cups; make a well in salsa with back of a spoon. Break 1 egg into each ramekin. Sprinkle 1 tablespoon cheese over each egg. Place in preheated oven. Bake 20 minutes or until eggs are set to your liking. Garnish each ramekin with a cilantro sprig. Makes 6 servings.

PER SERVING: 1/6 of total recipe

CALORIES	CARBOHYDRATES	PROTEIN	FAT	CHOLESTEROL
149	7 gm	9 gm	10 gm	286 mg

Quick Banana Milkshake

One banana a day gives you all the potassium you need. For a nutritious breakfast drink, use a frozen banana for a frosty milkshake instead of slicing it for cereal. Wrap peeled bananas in plastic wrap, then freeze. There's no need to thaw before slicing.

1 large banana, frozen (7 oz.)
1/2 cup plain low-fat yogurt
1/4 cup apple juice
1/2 cup unsweetened raspberries, boysenberries, strawberries
   or sliced peaches (fresh *or* frozen)

Slice banana. Place in blender container. Add yogurt and apple juice; process until thick and smooth. Add your choice of berries or fruit; puree. Pour into 4 glasses and serve immediately. Makes 4 (1/2-cup) servings.

PER SERVING: 1/2 cup

CALORIES	CARBOHYDRATES	PROTEIN	FAT	CHOLESTEROL
74	17 gm	2 gm	0 gm	0 mg

Creamy Tofu Cooler

One serving of this cooler supplies 20% of the US RDA for iron and 92% of the US RDA for vitamin C. The vitamin C enhances the absorption of the iron. Make the cooler with strawberries, bananas or blueberries, or combine all three for a star-spangled drink.

3/4 cup apple juice
1 teaspoon honey
2 oz. regular tofu, rinsed, drained
1/2 cup whole, hulled strawberries *or* 1 (3-inch) piece peeled
   banana *or* 1/4 cup blueberries (fresh *or* frozen)
2 ice cubes

In a blender, combine apple juice, honey, tofu and fruit. Process 30 seconds. Add ice cubes; process 20 seconds or until frothy. If using frozen blueberries, omit ice cubes. Makes 2 (1/2-cup) servings.

PER SERVING: 1/2 cup

CALORIES	CARBOHYDRATES	PROTEIN	FAT	CHOLESTEROL
119	26 gm	3 gm	1.5 gm	0 mg

Glossary

AEROBIC EXERCISE: Those types of physical activities that stimulate the heart and lungs for a sufficient amount of time to produce beneficial change in the body. Examples of aerobic exercise include running, cycling, crewing, cross-country running and skiing, swimming and aerobic dance.

BASAL METABOLIC RATE (BMR): The amount of energy required to sustain a person's minimal body functions—the energy it takes for you to blink your eyes and for your heart to beat.

CALORIE: A measure of a unit of heat or energy.

CHOLESTEROL: A waxy-like substance that is found in all animal fats, bile and brain tissue.

ELECTROLYTES: Electrically charged particles found in the body. They keep the chemical reactions of the body working properly.

ERGOGENIC AIDS: Substances which may enhance physical performance.

FATTY ACIDS: Components responsible for the different flavors, textures and melting points of fat. They can be saturated (of animal origin), polyunsaturated, or monosaturated (of plant origin).

FIBER: The part of food that is not digested by the body such as the seeds in a tomato.

GLUCOSE: Blood sugar—the simplest form of carbohydrate used for energy.

GLYCOGEN: The form that carbohydrate is stored in the body.

HYDROGENATION: A chemical process that turns an unsaturated fat into a saturated fat.

HYDROSTATIC WEIGHING: A technique used to assess percent body fat by weighing a person underwater.

LEGUMES: Plants that have edible seeds within a pod, such as peas, beans and lentils.

NUTRIENT: A substance needed by all living things to maintain life, health and reproduction.

OBESITY: A condition of carrying too much fat.

OVERFAT: A man is considered overfat if 15 percent or more of his total weight comes from fat. A woman is overfat if 22 percent or more of her total body weight is fat.

OVERWEIGHT: A term used to describe a person who weighs more than is recommended by the standard insurance height/weight charts.

PULSE OR HEART RATE: The number of times your heart beats in one minute.

RECOMMENDED DIETARY ALLOWANCES: The amount of various nutrients that a healthy person needs to maintain life processes.

UNITED STATES RECOMMENDED DAILY ALLOWANCE (US RDA): A tool developed by the Food and Drug Administration for food labeling. The US RDA represents the maximum amount of the RDA's for both males and females of all ages for each nutrient.

VEGETARIAN: A term that describes a person who does not eat animal products or who limits the types of animal products eaten.

Appendix

FOOD EXCHANGE LISTS

Each of the foods listed below is considered one "exchange." Each of the food items has about the same amount of carbohydrate (CHO), Protein (PRO), and Fat.

MEAT/FISH/POULTRY
Each exchange contains: CHO = 0 grams, PRO = 7 grams, FAT = 5 grams.

CHEESE:	1 ounce natural or processed cheese. One ounce is equivalent to 1″ cube.
	1/4 cup low-fat cottage cheese or grated brick cheese
	1 slice American cheese
EGG:	1 large
FISH:	1 ounce fish or shellfish, 5 small shrimp, clams or oysters
	1/4 cup flaked fish, such as canned tuna or canned salmon
MEAT:	1 ounce lean beef, lamb, pork or veal (10-15% fat)
PEANUT BUTTER:	2 tablespoons (peanut butter contains more fat than the other meat exchanges—2 tablespoons contain 14 gms.)

DAIRY PRODUCTS
Each exchange contains: CHO = 12 grams, PRO = 8 grams, FAT = 4 grams (maximum)

Milk:	1 cup low-fat or skim milk
	1 cup low-fat buttermilk
	1/4 cup nonfat dry milk powder
Other:	8 ounces low-fat yogurt

FRUIT
Each exchange contains: CHO = 10 grams, PRO = 0 grams, FAT = 0 grams.

Fresh Fruit:	1 small apple (2 inches in diameter)
	1/2 small banana
	1 cup berries (strawberries, raspberries, blackberries)
	2/3 cup blueberries
	1/4 cantaloupe (6 inches in diameter)
	10 sweet cherries
	2 dates or dried prunes
	2 tablespoons raisins
	1/2 small grapefruit
	1 small orange
	1/3 medium-size papaya
	1 medium-size peach
	1 small pear
	1 large tangerine
	1 cup cubed watermelon
	Canned fruit: 1/2 cup fruit packed in its own juice
Fruit juice:	1/3 cup apple juice
	1/2 cup orange juice, grapefruit juice, or pineapple juice
	1/4 cup sweetened cranberry juice; 1/2 cup unsweetened cranberry juice
	1/4 cup grape juice
	1/4 cup prune juice

BREADS & CEREALS
Each exchange contains: CHO = 15 grams, PRO = 2 grams, FAT = 0 grams

BREADS:	1 biscuit or muffin, 2-inch in diameter (contains added fat)
	1 bread slice, white or whole wheat
	2 "thin" bread slices
	1 small hamburger bun, hot dog bun, or dinner roll
	1/2 bagel or English muffin
	1 (6-inch) tortilla
	1 (4-inch) waffle or pancake (contains added fat)
CEREAL:	1 oz. ready-to-eat cereal (about 3/4 cup of most flaked cereals)
	1/2 cup cooked cereal
	2-2/3 tablespoons Grapenuts
	1/3 cup granola
	1 cup puffed cereal
CRACKERS:	2 (2-inch) square graham crackers
	5 saltines
	6 to 8 thin variety crackers (contain added fat)
PASTA/GRAINS:	1/2 cup cooked pasta:
	macaroni, spaghetti or noodles
	1/2 cup rice
VEGETABLES:	1/2 cup mashed potatoes
	1 (2-inch) baked potato
	1/2 cup cooked dried beans
	1/3 cup corn
	1/2 cup peas
OTHER:	10 to 15 potato or tortilla chips (about 5 grams of fat)
	1/2 cup ice cream (about 5 grams of fat)
	1 (2-inch) cookie (about 5 grams of fat)
	1 (2-inch) square of white cake (no icing)
	3 cups unbuttered popped popcorn
	6 (3-ring) pretzels
	1/3 cup sherbet

VEGETABLES
Each exchange contains: CHO = 5 grams, PRO = 2 grams, FAT = 0 grams. One exchange is equivalent to 1/2 cup of the following vegetables.

Artichoke	Eggplant
Asparagus	*Greens; lettuce, spinach, dandelion
Bean sprouts	greens, collard greens and turnip greens
Beans, wax or green	Red or green peppers
Broccoli	*Radishes
Brussel Sprouts	Sauerkraut
Cabbage	*Squash, summer
*Cauliflower	Tomatoes, tomato juice
*Celery	Mushrooms
*Cucumbers	Okra
Onions	Parsley

*These vegetables are considered "free" for a person who is watching his weight. In other words these vegetables can be eaten in unlimited amounts.

FATS
Each exchange contains: CHO = 0 grams, PRO = 0 grams, FAT = 5 grams.

1/8th of a medium-size avocado
2 teaspoons reduced-calorie margarine
1 slice bacon
1 teaspoon chocolate (unsweetened)
2 tablespoons grated coconut
2 tablespoons cream, light or sour
2 tablespoons whipped cream
1 tablespoon cream cheese
2 tablespoons lite cream cheese
1 teaspoon mayonnaise
1 tablespoon light mayonnaise
1 teaspoon oil
5 small olives

Nuts: 10 almonds   12 peanuts
      2 brazil nuts   6 walnut or pecan halves
      7 cashews   20 Pistachios
      3 macadamia

1 tablespoon salad dressing (Blue Cheese, French, Italian, Thousand Island)
1 teaspoon shortening
2 teaspoons tartar sauce

ADDRESSES FOR FAST FOOD RESTAURANTS

ARBY'S
Ten Piedmont Ctr.
3495 Piedmont Rd. N.E.
Atlanta, GA 30305

BURGER CHEF
College Park Pyramids
P.O. Box 927
Indianapolis, IN 46206

BURGER KING
P.O. Box 520783
General Mail Facility
Miami, FL 33152

CHURCH'S FRIED CHICKEN
P.O. Box BH001
San Antonio, TX 78284

HARDEE'S
1233 N. Church Street
Rocky Mount, NC 27801

JACK IN THE BOX
Foodmaker, Inc.
9330 Balboa Ave.
San Diego, CA 92123

KENTUCKY FRIED CHICKEN
P.O. Box 32070
Louisville, KY 90232

LONG JOHN SILVER'S
P.O. Box 11988
Lexington, KY 40579

McDONALD'S
McDonald's Plaza
Oak Brook, IL 60521

PIZZA HUT
P.O. Box 428
Wichita, KS 97201

WENDY'S
9288 W. Dublin
Dublin, OH 43017

VITAMINS & MINERALS

VITAMIN/MINERAL	FUNCTION	FOOD SOURCE
VITAMIN A	Promotes healthy skin, hair and mucous membranes. Necessary for good night vision, normal reproduction and proper development of bones and teeth. Helps the body absorb calcium and phosphorus.	Carrots, broccoli, spinach, liver, egg yolk, milk and dairy products.
VITAMIN D	Builds strong bones and teeth. Helps the body absorb calcium and phosphorus.	Fish, eggs, milk and it is manufactured in the skin with exposure to sunlight.
VITAMIN E	Helps in the formation of red blood cells, muscles and other tissues. Protects vitamins A and C and essential fatty acids from destruction.	Green leafy vegetables, vegetable oil, whole-grain cereals, bread and liver.
VITAMIN K	Helps produce the substances that make blood clot.	Cabbage, Brussels sprouts, kale and milk.
THIAMIN (B_1)	Promotes the release of energy from carbohydrates, helps synthesize nerve-regulating substances.	Pork, liver, oysters, cereals, nuts and legumes.
RIBOFLAVIN (B_2)	Helps release energy from carbohydrate, proteins and fats. Maintains skin and eye tissue.	Dark green vegetables, whole grains, pasta, mushrooms, milk, eggs, meat and fish.
NIACIN (B_3)	Works with thiamin and riboflavin in energy production within the cells.	Poultry, meat, fish, tuna, peanut butter, dried peas and beans.
PYRIDOXINE (B_6)	Needed to build genetic material and aids in the functioning of the nervous system.	Kidney, meat, fish, eggs, milk and oysters.
B_{12}	Helps in the formation of red blood cells and aids in the building of genetic material, assists in the functioning of the nervous system.	Liver, kidney, meat, fish, eggs, milk and oysters.
PANTOTHENIC ACID	Assists in the metabolism of carbohydrates, protein and fats, and in the formation of hormones and nerve regulating substances.	Kidney, liver, whole-grain breads and cereals, nuts, eggs and dark green vegetables.
BIOTIN	Helps release energy from carbohydrates and assists in the formation of fatty acids.	Liver, kidneys, egg yolk, dark green vegetables and green beans.

VITAMINS & MINERALS (continued)

VITAMIN/MINERAL	FUNCTION	FOOD SOURCE
FOLACIN	Works with vitamin B_{12} to synthesize red blood cells, helps in the formation of hemoglobin in red blood cells.	Dark green leafy vegetables, fruits and soybeans.
VITAMIN C	Helps maintain bones, teeth and blood vessels. Helps protect other vitamins from oxidation—may help block the formation of cancer-causing substances.	Citrus fruits, strawberries, tomatoes, melons, green pepper and potatoes.
CALCIUM	Helps build strong bones and teeth. Participates in muscle contraction, blood clotting and nerve conduction.	Milk, cheese, small fish eaten with the bones, dried peas, beans and dark green leafy vegetables.
PHOSPHORUS	Works with calcium to promote strong bones and teeth. Needed for metabolism of fats and carbohydrates.	Liver, kidney, meat, fish, eggs, milk and dairy products, nuts and legumes.
CHLORINE	Helps produce gastric juices and participates in the digestive process.	Table salt
ZINC	Constituent of many enzymes which enable the body to grow and function properly.	Liver, meat, eggs, poultry, seafood, whole grain breads and dairy products.
MAGNESIUM	Helps regulate body temperature. Participates in nerve and muscle contraction and protein synthesis. Activates enzymes for carbohydrate metabolism.	Green leafy vegetables, whole grains, nuts and beans.
SODIUM	Regulates water balance, muscle contraction, and nerve conduction.	Salt, salted foods, soy sauce, MSG, baking powder, cheese, fish, poultry, eggs.
POTASSIUM	Works with sodium to promote fluid balance, helps regulate heartbeat.	Fresh fruit, dark green vegetables, potatoes with skin, liver, meat, fish, poultry, milk.
IRON	Part of the hemoglobin in the blood. Transports and transfers oxygen in the blood and tissues.	Liver, eggs, legumes, lean meat, whole grains, green leafy vegetables, enriched cereals.
SULFUR	Helps build proteins such as hair, nails and cartilage.	Eggs, meat, milk, cheese, nuts, legumes.

RECOMMENDED DAILY DIETARY ALLOWANCES, REVISED 1980

Designed for the Maintenance of Good Nutrition of Practically All Healthy People in the U.S.A.[a]

	AGE (yrs)	WT. (kgs)	WT. (lbs)	HT. (cm)	HT. (in)	PRO-TEIN (g)	VIT. A (RE)[b]	VIT. D (μg)[c]	VIT. E (mg)[d]	VIT. C (mg)	THIA-MIN (mg)	RIBO FLAVIN (mg)	NIACIN (mg NE)[e]	VIT. B6 (mg)	FOLA-CIN (μg)	VIT. B12 (μg)	CALCIUM (mg)	PHOS-PHO-RUS (mg)	MAG-NE-SIUM (mg)	IRON (mg)	ZINC (mg)	IODINE (μg)
Males	11-14	45	99	157	62	45	1000	10	8	50	1.4	1.6	18	1.8	400	3.0	1200	1200	350	18	15	150
	15-18	66	145	176	69	56	1000	10	10	60	1.4	1.7	18	2.0	400	3.0	1200	1200	400	18	15	150
	19-22	70	154	177	70	56	1000	7.5	10	60	1.5	1.7	19	2.2	400	3.0	800	800	350	10	15	150
	23-50	70	154	178	70	56	1000	5	10	60	1.4	1.6	18	2.2	400	3.0	800	800	350	10	15	150
	51+	70	154	178	70	56	1000	5	10	60	1.2	1.4	16	2.2	400	3.0	800	800	350	10	15	150
Females	11-14	46	101	157	62	46	800	10	8	50	1.1	1.3	15	1.8	400	3.0	1200	1200	300	18	15	150
	15-18	55	120	163	64	46	800	10	8	60	1.1	1.3	14	2.0	400	3.0	1200	1200	300	18	15	150
	19-22	55	120	163	64	44	800	7.5	8	60	1.1	1.3	14	2.0	400	3.0	800	800	300	18	15	150
	23-50	55	120	163	64	44	800	5	8	60	1.0	1.2	13	2.0	400	3.0	800	800	300	18	15	150
	51+	55	120	163	64	44	800	5	8	60	1.0	1.2	13	2.0	400	3.0	800	800	300	10	15	150
Pregnant						+30	+200	+5	+2	+20	+0.4	+0.3	+2	+0.6	+400	+1.0	+400	+400	+150	f	+5	+25
Lactating						+20	+400	+5	+3	+40	+0.5	+0.5	+5	+0.5	+100	+1.0	+400	+400	+150	18	+10	+50

a   The allowances are intended to provide for individual variations among most normal persons as they live in the United States under usual environmental stresses. Diets should be based on a variety of common foods in order to provide other nutrients for which human requirements have been less well defined.

b   Retinol equivalents. 1 retinol equivalent = 1 μg retinol or 6 μg β carotene.

c   As cholecalciferol. 10 μg cholecalciferol = 400 IU of vitamin D.

d   α-tocopherol equivalents. 1 mg d-α-tocopherol = 1 TE

e   1 NE (niacin equivalent) is equal to 1 mg of niacin or 60 mg of dietary tryptophan.

f   30 to 60mg of supplemental iron is needed in addition to dietary intake.

Reproduced from National Academy of Sciences: Recommended Dietary Allowances, 9th rev. ed. Washington, D.C. 1980.

Index